Introduction to Pharmaceutical Calculations

D1319531

Introduction to Pharmaceutical Calculations

Judith A Rees
BPharm, MSc, PhD, MRPharmS

Senior Lecturer
School of Pharmacy and Pharmaceutical Sciences
University of Manchester, UK

Ian Smith
BSc, MRPharmS

Boots Teacher Practitioner
School of Pharmacy and Pharmaceutical Sciences
University of Manchester, UK

Brian Smith
BSc(Hons), MSc

Formerly Mathematics Teacher
Manchester, UK

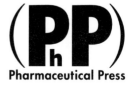

Pharmaceutical Press

Published by the Pharmaceutical Press
1 Lambeth High Street, London SE1 7JN, UK

First published 2001

© Pharmaceutical Press 2001

Text design by Barker/Hilsdon, Lyme Regis, Dorset
Typeset by Type Study, Scarborough, North Yorkshire
Printed in Great Britain by TJ International, Padstow, Cornwall

ISBN 0 85369 449 4

A catalogue record for this book is available from the British Library

"No man dies until he is forgotten"

We would like to dedicate this book to the memory of Brian Smith who died suddenly on 11 March 2000. Without his ideas related to the teaching and learning of mathematics this book would not and could not have happened. He will be greatly missed by his wife and children, his grandchildren and everyone who knew him.

Contents

Preface   x
Acknowledgement   xii
About the authors   xiii

1   **Rational numbers**   1
     Proportional sets of numbers   1
     Ratios   3
     Fractions   3
     Decimals   7
     Percentages   8
     Accuracy of measurement   9
     Finding a missing value from two proportional sets   14
     Setting up proportional sets for practical situations   21
     Proportional sets that become trivial   24
     Practice calculations   25
     Answers   29

2   **Systems of units**   33
     Mass and weight   33
     Metric units   33
     Changing metric units   34
     Changing units between different systems of measurement   36
     Conversions of temperature between degrees Fahrenheit
        and degrees Celsius   37
     Practice calculations   40
     Answers   41

3   **Concentrations**   43
     Introduction   43
     Amount strengths   44
     Ratio strengths   45
     Parts per million   47
     Percentage concentration   49

Converting expressions of concentration from one form
  to another   49
Calculating the amount of ingredient required to make up
  a percentage solution   54
Calculating the amount of ingredient required to prepare
  a ratio strength solution   55
Practice calculations   56
Answers   58

4   Dilutions   61
Simple dilutions   61
Serial dilutions   63
Concentrated waters   66
Triturations   68
Powder calculations   70
Multiple dilutions   75
Mixing concentrations   81
Practice calculations   86
Answers   88

5   Formulations   91
Reducing the formula   91
Increasing the formula   93
Formulae involving parts   94
Formulae containing percentages   97
Practice calculations   99
Answers   102

6   Calculation of doses   105
Definition of dose and dosage regimen   105
Doses based on units of formulations   106
Doses based on the weight of drug   110
Doses based on body weight   113
Doses based on body surface area   118
Doses as a percentage of the adult dose   120
Doses based on units   121
Practice calculations   122
Answers   127

7   Displacement volumes and values, and density   131
Displacement volumes involving solids in liquids   131
Displacement values involving solids incorporated
  into other solids   136
Density   143

Practice calculations   146
Answers   149

8   Calculations involving molecular weights   151
Molecular weights of drugs   151
Calculation of legal classifications using molecular weights   161
Moles and millimoles   165
Molar solutions   169
Milliequivalents   173
Practice calculations   175
Answers   177

9   Parenteral solutions and isotonicity   179
Rate of flow of intravenous solutions   179
Isotonicity   188
Practice calculations   190
Answers   193

Bibliography   195

Appendix: Atomic weights of the elements   197

Index   200

Preface

In teaching pharmacy practice it has become apparent that many students, even those with an A level in mathematics, encounter difficulties in performing pharmaceutical calculations. The difficulties do not seem to disappear on graduation and many pre-registration students encounter problems with pharmaceutical calculations. Since any calculation error may potentially harm or even lead to the death of a patient it is vitally important, particularly in this litigious age, that pharmacists and other healthcare professionals are able to carry out calculations with confidence.

There seems to be a need for a textbook that will support the teaching of pharmaceutical calculations and form a reference source for busy practising pharmacists and other healthcare professionals. In producing this book, the help of an experienced teacher of mathematics has been enlisted and he was able to show that almost all pharmaceutical calculations could be dealt with by a single approach. Traditionally, different types of questions seem to have been tackled by different methods and students have found particular difficulties in deciding the order in which pieces of information given in the question should be used. In the approach used in this book, the first step is for the user to organise given and required data from a question into proportional sets. The second step is to apply some simple algebra to find the required unknown value. A third step (not necessary but highly recommended) is the placing of the calculated result back into the proportional sets where it becomes apparent whether or not the calculated result is of about the correct size, thus giving an important extra accuracy check.

The first two chapters of the book introduce the user to this novel, proportional sets approach, to the basic mathematical concepts on which it depends and also to systems of units and conversion between units. In the rest of the book the approach is applied to examples in the following pharmacy topics:

- concentrations
- simple and serial dilutions of solids and liquids

- multiple dilutions involving more than one expression of concentration
- reduction and enlargement of formulae for pharmaceutical products
- calculations involving concentrated waters and flavours
- doses and dosage regimens
- displacement values and volumes
- density
- molecular weight
- parenteral injections
- isotonicity.

The book has been designed so that the reader can use the text either to support learning or as a reference source to check understanding. Throughout the book worked examples are clearly laid out and practice calculations with answers are provided at the end of each chapter.

Overall we have tried to design this book so that it presents pharmaceutical calculations in a clear and consistent way. Hopefully, pharmacy students, pharmacists and other healthcare professionals will no longer have difficulties with calculations and ultimately the patient will be safer.

Judith A Rees, Ian Smith, Brian Smith
Manchester, 2000

Acknowledgement

We wish to express our indebtedness to the late Richard Skemp on whose work the proportional sets approach to rational numbers used in this book is based.

About the authors

Judith A Rees studied pharmacy in Bradford before completing a PhD in Manchester. She is currently a senior lecturer in the School of Pharmacy and Pharmaceutical Sciences at the University of Manchester, where she teaches in the area of pharmacy practice.

Ian Smith studied pharmacy in Manchester. He is a Boots Teacher Practitioner, which combines being a pharmacist with Boots the Chemists and teaching pharmacy practice in the School of Pharmacy and Pharmaceutical Sciences at the University of Manchester.

Brian Smith studied mathematics at Manchester University before completing an MSc in computer-aided engineering. He taught mathematics in grammar schools and in a sixth-form college. He was an examiner in mathematics up to 'A' level for the Northern Examinations and Assessment Board.

1

Rational numbers

Most students will already have at least a basic knowledge of arithmetic and algebra, so the aim of this chapter is to provide a reinforcement of the particular mathematical concepts that are necessary in order to carry out the calculations required in Pharmacy. School mathematics courses tend to treat the basic tools of fractions, decimals and percentages as quite separate topics. In this book an attempt is made to provide a more unified and hopefully a more interesting approach.

Proportional sets of numbers

Consider the following sets of data.
A drug is in solution at a concentration of 75 mg to 5 mL:

weight of drug (mg)	15	30	45	60	75	90 ...
volume of solution (mL)	1	2	3	4	5	6 ...

A heavy vehicle travels at a steady speed of 15 miles per hour:

distance travelled (miles)	15	30	45	60	75	90 ...
time taken (hours)	1	2	3	4	5	6 ...

In these two sets of data we see that the numbers are the same. The same arrangement of numbers serves as an image for two quite different practical situations.

Let us extract the two sets of numbers:

set A	15	30	45	60	75	90 ...
set B	1	2	3	4	5	6 ...

We see that there is a relationship between the two sets: each number in set A is 15 times the corresponding number in set B.

When one set of numbers is obtained by multiplying each number of the other set by a fixed number, the two sets are said to be *proportional*. Thus we can say that set A is proportional to set B.

Now consider the next two sets of numbers:

3   5   9 . . .

12   20   36 . . .

In this example each lower number is obtained by multiplying the corresponding upper number by 4. Again the two sets are proportional.

Now consider the next two sets of numbers:

3   8   13   18 . . .

1   2   3   4 . . .

There is no fixed number by which the lower set of values can be multiplied in order to arrive at corresponding values of the upper set or vice versa. The two sets are not proportional to each other.

EXAMPLES 1.1–1.5
_____

In each of the following questions decide whether or not the pairs of sets are proportional.

1.1   *6   10   14*

         3   5   7

Proportional. Each value of the upper set is twice the corresponding value of the lower set.

1.2   *5   7   9*

         40   56   72

Proportional. Each value of the lower set is eight times the corresponding value of the upper set.

1.3   *2   4   8*

         1   2   3

Not proportional.

1.4   *5   7   9*

         15   17   19

Not proportional.

1.5   *16   17   21*

        80   85   105

Proportional. Each value of the lower set is five times the corresponding value of the upper set.

Ratios

Proportional sets can be used to explain the term 'ratio'.

For the proportional sets:

   9   21   30   36 . . .

   3   7   10   12 . . .

each number in the upper set is three times the corresponding number in the lower set. Each of the corresponding pairs of numbers is said to be in the ratio three to one.

For the next pair of proportional sets:

   2   5   7 . . .

  10   25   35 . . .

one to five is the ratio of the corresponding pairs. The ratio one to five can also be expressed as 1:5.

Numbers that represent ratios are called *rational numbers*. Fractions, decimals and percentages are three kinds of numerals that can be used to represent rational numbers. We will examine the relationships between these three different notations.

Fractions

The ratio 4 to 1 is represented by the fraction $\frac{4}{1}$, which is equivalent to the natural number 4. (The *natural numbers* are the counting numbers 1, 2, 3, . . .)

The ratio 1 to 5 is represented by the fraction $\frac{1}{5}$. The number on top of a fraction is called the numerator and the bottom number is the denominator:

$$\text{fraction} = \frac{\text{numerator}}{\text{denominator}}$$

Consider the proportional sets:

1   2   3   4 . . .

5   10   15   20 . . .

We can see that ratio 1 to 5 = ratio 2 to 10 = ratio 3 to 15 and so on. Since each ratio can be represented by a fraction, we can write down as many different names as we wish for any given fraction:

$$\frac{1}{5} = \frac{2}{10} = \frac{3}{15} = \frac{4}{20} = \frac{5}{25} \text{ and so on.}$$

To obtain other names for a given fraction we multiply (or divide) both numerator and denominator by the same number.

EXAMPLE 1.6
_____

Find the numerator of the fraction that is equal to $\frac{1}{7}$ but has denominator 21.

Let the numerator be x:

$$\frac{1}{7} = \frac{x}{21}$$

Denominator 7 has been multiplied by 3 to get new denominator 21, so numerator 1 must be multiplied by 3 to get x, therefore $x = 3$.
    The numerator is 3.

EXAMPLE 1.7
_____

Find the numerator of the fraction that is equal to $\frac{16}{24}$ but has denominator 3.

Let the numerator be y:

$$\frac{y}{3} = \frac{16}{24}$$

Denominator 24 has been divided by 8 to get new denominator 3, so numerator 16 must be divided by 8 to get y, therefore $y = 2$.

The numerator is 2.

EXAMPLE 1.8

Find the denominator of the fraction that is equal to $\frac{80}{180}$ but has numerator 16.

Let the denominator be x:

$$\frac{16}{x} = \frac{80}{180}$$

Numerator 80 has been divided by 5 to get 16, so x is 180 divided by 5, therefore $x = 36$.

The denominator is 36.

Fractions expressed in their lowest terms

Since there are many names for the same fraction, the one we tend to use to represent the fraction is the one for which there is no whole number that will divide exactly into both the numerator and the denominator. The fraction is then said to be expressed in its lowest terms.

EXAMPLE 1.9

Express $\frac{35}{45}$ in its lowest terms.

Both 35 and 45 can be divided by 5. We divide numerator and denominator by 5 to get $\frac{7}{9}$.

EXAMPLE 1.10

Express $\frac{60}{405}$ in its lowest terms.

We can see that 60 and 405 will divide by 5, so

$$\frac{60}{405} = \frac{12}{81}$$

Now 12 and 81 will divide by 3, so

$$\frac{60}{405} = \frac{12}{81} = \frac{4}{27}$$

Multiplication of a fraction by a whole number

We have seen that if both the numerator and the denominator of a fraction are multiplied by the same number the resulting fraction is equal to the first one and is just another name for it. To multiply a fraction by a whole number (an *integer*) we multiply only the numerator by the integer. Thus:

$\frac{4}{7}$ multiplied by 3 becomes $\frac{12}{7}$

$\frac{5}{9}$ multiplied by 7 becomes $\frac{35}{9}$

When $\frac{6}{7}$ is multiplied by 8 the result is $\frac{48}{7}$, which can be written as $\frac{42}{7} + \frac{6}{7}$ = $6\frac{6}{7}$.

Decimals

In the number 127, the 1 represents one hundred, the 2 represents two tens and the 7 represents seven units. The value of each digit is therefore dependent on its position in the number. This system of 'place values' is extended for the representation of decimals by introducing a decimal point after the unit value.

Units		Tenths	Hundredths	Thousandths	Ten-thousandths
0	.	2	3		
0	.	5	2		7

The number 0.23 is a rational number. The 2 is in the tenths column and the 3 is in the hundredths column. Two tenths and three hundredths make twenty-three hundredths, so 0.23 is another name for the fraction $\frac{23}{100}$.

The number 0.527 has a 7 in the thousandths column so it is another name for the fraction $\frac{527}{1000}$.

For the reverse process, i.e. to express a fraction in decimal form, the numerator is simply divided by the denominator:

$$\frac{24}{64} = 24 \text{ divided by } 64 = 0.375.$$

Note that $\frac{2}{5}, \frac{4}{10}$ and $\frac{6}{15}$ are different names for the same fraction. Changing each fraction to a decimal:

2 divided by 5 = 4 divided by 10 = 3 divided by 15 = 0.4.

Thus one decimal may be represented by many fractions.

EXAMPLE 1.11

Convert 0.3 to a fraction.

The 3 is in the tenths column so $0.3 = \frac{3}{10}$.

EXAMPLE 1.12

Convert 0.35 to a fraction.

The 5 is in the hundredths column so $0.35 = \frac{35}{100} = \frac{7}{20}$.

EXAMPLE 1.13

Convert the fraction $\frac{3}{5}$ to a decimal.

3 divided by 5 gives 0.6
or

$$\frac{3}{5} = \frac{6}{10} = 0.6$$

EXAMPLE 1.14

Convert the fraction $\frac{7}{8}$ to a decimal.

7 divided by 8 gives 0.875.

Percentages

5 per cent means 5 per hundred, so 5% represents the same rational number as the fraction

$$\frac{5}{100} = \frac{5}{5 \times 20} = \frac{1}{20}$$

Similarly, 31% is the same as $\frac{31}{100}$.

To change a fraction to a percentage, we can change the fraction to a decimal and then examine the decimal to see how many units there are in the hundredths column. The number of hundredths gives the percentage. For example, let us convert the fraction $\frac{1}{20}$ to a percentage. First divide 1 by 20 to get the decimal 0.05. There is a 5 in the hundredths column. Five hundredths is equal to 5%.

Similarly, the fraction $\frac{3}{40}$ = 3 divided by 40 = 0.075. There is a 7 in the hundredths column, so there are 7.5 hundredths, which is 7.5%.

EXAMPLE 1.15

Express 0.76 as a percentage.

There is a 6 in the hundredths column:

0.76 = 76 hundredths = 76%

EXAMPLE 1.16

Express 0.769 as a percentage.

There is a 6 in the hundredths column:

0.769 = 76.9 hundredths = 76.9%

EXAMPLE 1.17
_____

Express 20% as a fraction in its lowest terms.

$$20\% = \frac{20}{100} = \frac{1}{5}$$

EXAMPLE 1.18
_____

Express 0.2% as a fraction in its lowest terms.

$$0.2\% = \frac{0.2}{100} = \frac{2}{1000} = \frac{1}{500}$$

EXAMPLE 1.19
_____

Express $\frac{7}{10}$ as a percentage.

$$\frac{7}{10} = 0.70 = 70\%$$

EXAMPLE 1.20
_____

Express $\frac{3}{8}$ as a percentage.

$$\frac{3}{8} = 0.375 = 37.5\%$$

Accuracy of measurement

Consider the following statement:

The room is 15.342 metres long.

In the 15.342 metres, the last figure 2 is in the millimetre column so the length in millimetres is 15342. It is unlikely that anyone would want to know the length of a room to that degree of accuracy and it is also unlikely that the measurement could be made to that degree of accuracy. The figure 2 is not only unnecessary but may also be misleading, implying that the measurement is more accurate than it really is.

Significant figures

If the room were measured to the nearest centimetre, the result would be 1534 centimetres. Its length to the nearest metre would be 15 metres. Converting this to centimetres gives a length of 1500 centimetres. In this number, the 1 means one thousand, the 5 means five hundreds, but the 00 does not mean 0 tens and 0 units. The 00 means that the number of tens and the number of units are not stated. The zeros are there to act as spacers so that the 1 appears in the thousands column and the 5 appears in the hundreds column. Since the 1 and the 5 mean what they say, they are *significant figures*. The two zeros are not significant figures.

EXAMPLE 1.21

A bottle contains 60 mL of a liquid to the nearest 10 mL. How many significant figures are there?

The 6 means 6 tens but the 0 means that the number of units is not stated. There is one significant figure.

EXAMPLE 1.22

A bottle contains 0.04 L of a liquid to the nearest 0.01 L. How many significant figures are there?

The number 0.04 can be written as 0.040. The 0 to the right of the 4 means that the number of thousandths of a litre is unknown and it and any more zeros that may be written to the right of it are not significant. The 4 means 4 hundredths of a litre and is significant. The 0 to the left of the 4 appears only as a spacer to make the 4 appear in the hundredths column so it is not significant. There is one significant figure.

EXAMPLE 1.23

The number 152 000 is stated to the nearest hundred. How many significant figures are there?

The 0 after the 2 means that there are no hundreds. The following 00 means that the number of tens and the number of units are not stated. There are four significant figures.

Note: If a number is stated in the form 0.340 (rather than 0.34) and we are not told to what degree of accuracy the number is stated, the zero to the right of the 4 would be interpreted as indicating that there are no thousandths and that the number was correct to the nearest thousandth. There would be three significant figures.

Correcting to fewer significant figures

In order to correct 33.62 to *two* significant figures, we consider the first *three* significant figures. 33.6 is closer to 34 than it is to 33 so 33.62 corrected to two significant figures is 34.

In order to correct 33.42 to *two* significant figures, we consider the first *three* significant figures. 33.4 is closer to 33 than it is to 34 so 33.42 corrected to two significant figures is 33.

Note: In order to correct 33.52 to *two* significant figures, we consider the first *three* significant figures. We regard 33.5 as being closer to 34 than it is to 33 so 33.52 corrected to two significant figures is 34.

EXAMPLES 1.24–1.27

1.24 *Correct 17586 to three significant figures.*   Answer 17600
1.25 *Correct 17536 to three significant figures.*   Answer 17500
1.26 *Correct 0.0003274 to two significant figures.*   Answer 0.00033
1.27 *Correct 0.0003234 to two significant figures.*   Answer 0.00032

Correcting to a certain number of decimal places

The method used is similar to that used to deal with correction to a certain number of significant figures.

Look at the figure in the column to the right of the last decimal place required. If the figure is 4 or less, it and any digits to the right of it are deleted. If the digit is a 5 or higher, the digit of the last decimal place is increased by 1 and any digits to the right are deleted.

EXAMPLES 1.28–1.31

1.28 Correct 1.5654 to three decimal places.   Answer 1.565
1.29 Correct 1.5655 to three decimal places.   Answer 1.566
1.30 Correct 21.7234 to two decimal places.   Answer 21.72
1.31 Correct 21.7258 to two decimal places.   Answer 21.73

Accuracy in arithmetic calculations

If all the values involved in a calculation are exact then it will be possible to calculate the exact value of the result. If, however, some of the values involved in a calculation are inexact and have been stated to a certain number of significant figures, a decision needs to be made as to how many figures of the result are likely to be significant. The following rough and ready rule may provide some help in cases in which the arithmetic operations involved are multiplication and division. The rule is find the value involved in the calculation which has the least number of significant figures and correct the result to that number of significant figures.

The user should, however, be aware that the actual number of reliable significant figures could be even smaller. In cases involving addition and subtraction, only the least number of decimal places should be retained. Throughout a calculation, numbers should be retained to more significant figures than those required in the final result and correcting to the required number of significant figures should only be carried out at the end of the calculation.

Errors built up in arithmetic calculations

When, because of measuring difficulties, numbers are stated as estimates to a certain number of significant figures, errors are introduced. Further errors are built up when calculations are carried out and if there is a need to keep a close check on the extent of the errors it is possible to do so by finding lower and upper bounds for the possible values of the result.

As an example of this approach, consider the expression:

$$\frac{21.3 \times 124.6}{32.4}$$

where each number is stated correct to one decimal place.

21.349 corrected to three significant figures becomes 21.3

21.312 corrected to three significant figures becomes 21.3

21.273 corrected to three significant figures becomes 21.3

21.251 corrected to three significant figures becomes 21.3

Thus, we can see that any number in the interval from 21.25 to 21.35 (but not including the number 21.35) will be represented by the number 21.3 after correction to three significant figures. The number 21.3 represents any number in the interval from 21.25 to 21.35, so in using 21.3 there is a possible error of up to 0.05. Similarly, 124.6 represents any number in the interval from 124.55 to 124.65 and 32.4 represents any number in the interval from 32.35 to 32.45.

When 21.3 is multiplied by 124.6, the smallest value that can be obtained is the one achieved by multiplying the *smallest* value represented by 21.3 by the *smallest* value represented by 124.6, i.e. 21.25 × 124.55, giving 2646.6875. The smallest value of the result will be obtained by dividing 2646.6875 by the *largest* value represented by 32.4, i.e. 32.45, giving 81.562018.

When 21.3 is multiplied by 124.6, the largest value that can be obtained is the one achieved by multiplying the *largest* value represented by 21.3 by the *largest* value represented by 124.6, i.e. 21.35 × 124.65, giving 2661.2775. The largest value of the result will be obtained by dividing 2661.2775 by the *smallest* value represented by 32.4, i.e. 32.35, giving 82.265147.

We have found lower and upper limits of 81.562018 and 82.265147 for the result of the calculation. Using a calculator to evaluate the expression, the result is 81.912963. Each of these three values becomes 82 when corrected to two significant figures. Applying the rule stated above (p. 12), values 21.3 and 32.4 are those involved in the calculation which have the least number of significant figures. Correcting the calculator result to the same number of significant figures gives 81.9, but we see that there is a possible error of about 0.35, so the third figure is in doubt. This supports the warning expressed earlier that the actual number of reliable significant figures may be smaller than that provided by the rule.

Finding a missing value from two proportional sets

Most of the calculations encountered in dispensing are dependent on being able to find missing values from sets of proportional numbers and we are now almost ready to tackle the method for doing this. We have looked at the different forms of rational numbers such as fractions, decimals and percentages that may be required in carrying out the tasks. (We have not dealt with methods of adding or multiplying fractions because, if a calculator is available, it is usually easier to carry out these operations after converting the fractions to decimals.)

We need one more piece of work before we can proceed. Consider the following two proportional sets:

$$\text{set A} \quad p \quad q$$
$$\text{set B} \quad r \quad s$$

Let us take the sets formed by the values in the vertical columns and call them set C and set D. Thus we have:

$$\text{set C} \quad p \quad r$$
$$\text{set D} \quad q \quad s$$

As set A is proportional to set B, then we have learned that the ratio of p to r is equal to the ratio of q to s and this can be expressed as:

$$\frac{p}{r} = \frac{q}{s}$$

Multiplying both sides of the equation by rs gives:

$$ps = rq$$

Dividing both sides of this equation by qs gives:

$$\frac{p}{q} = \frac{r}{s}$$

This means that set C is proportional to set D.

Let us now re-state this important result:

	set C	set D
set A	p	q
set B	r	s

If set A is proportional to set B, then set C is proportional to set D.
Let us check the result with a specific example:

set A	2	10
set B	4	20

Each value of set B is twice the corresponding value of set A, so set A is proportional to set B.
Interchanging the horizontal and vertical columns:

set C	2	4
set D	10	20

Each value of set D is five times the corresponding value of set C, so set C is proportional to set D.

In finding missing numbers from proportional sets we will consider three methods and denote them method A, method B and method C. Method A is the general method, which can be used in all cases. Methods B and C are only applicable to a limited number of cases, but in such cases they will provide a simpler approach.

EXAMPLE 1.32
_____

For the proportional sets:

7   *y*   9   *10* . . .

21   24   27   30 . . .

find the missing value y.

Method A

We set up an equation using the value *y* and its corresponding value 24 along with any other corresponding pair. Corresponding pairs of values are in the same ratio so:

$$\frac{y}{24} = \frac{9}{27}$$

The value of the variable y will remain unchanged if both sides of this equation are multiplied by a constant. We multiply both sides of the equation by 24 to get rid of the fraction involving y:

$$24 \times \frac{y}{24} = 24 \times \frac{9}{27}$$

Multiplying the fractions by the whole numbers (see p. 6):

$$\frac{24y}{24} = \frac{216}{27}$$

This simplifies to give $y = 8$.

Note: This is the general method, which can be applied to any pair of proportional sets.

This example also lends itself to solution by method B.

Method B

In this method we 'spot' the relationship between the proportional sets. Each value of the lower set is three times the corresponding value of the upper set, so y times 3 = 24, therefore $y = 8$.

Method B is the easier method to apply in the limited number of cases in which it is applicable.

EXAMPLE 1.33

For the proportional sets:

x	*14*
25	*50*

find the missing number x.

If we attempt to use method B, we find that there is no obvious number that 50 can be divided by to get 14, but we are able to apply method C.

Method C

From the result on p. 15, the two vertical sets of numbers are proportional. The ratio of 50 to 25 is 2, so the ratio of 14 to x is also 2.

14 is divided by 2 to give $x = 7$. Again we are able to 'spot' the answer.

Method A

Corresponding pairs of values are in the same ratio so:

$$\frac{x}{25} = \frac{14}{50}$$

The value of the variable x will remain unchanged if both sides of this equation are multiplied by a constant. We multiply both sides of the equation by 25 to get rid of the fraction involving x:

$$25 \times \frac{x}{25} = 25 \times \frac{14}{50}$$

$$\frac{25x}{25} = \frac{350}{50}$$

This simplifies to give $x = 7$.

EXAMPLE 1.34

For the proportional sets:

3	x
5	8

find the missing value x.

Method A is the more appropriate method this time. Corresponding pairs are in the same ratio, so

$$\frac{x}{8} = \frac{3}{5}$$

Multiplying both sides of the equation by 8:

$$\frac{8 \times x}{8} = \frac{3 \times 8}{5}$$

$$x = \frac{24}{5}$$

The missing value is four and four fifths = 4.8.

Note: If this example is compared with Example 1.33 method A, we can see that this time a step has been missed out. Now that we understand what is happening in solving the algebraic fractional equation, we can probably miss out yet another step and go directly from

$$\frac{x}{8} = \frac{3}{5}$$

to

$$x = \frac{24}{5}$$

We will use this in Example 1.35.

EXAMPLE 1.35

For the pair of proportional sets:

z	9
6	15

find the missing value z.

Using method A, corresponding pairs of values are in the same ratio, so:

$$\frac{z}{6} = \frac{9}{15}$$

$$z = \frac{54}{15}$$

$$z = 3.6$$

EXAMPLE 1.36

For the proportional sets:

37	52
7	z

find the missing number z.

Using method A, corresponding pairs of values are in the same ratio, so we could write:

$$\frac{37}{7} = \frac{52}{z}$$

It would, however, make the fractional equation easier to solve if we were to write down the equivalent equation:

$$\frac{z}{52} = \frac{7}{37}$$

Then

$$z = \frac{364}{37}$$

$$z = 9.837837\ldots$$

Correcting to three significant figures gives $z = 9.84$.

EXAMPLE 1.37

Consider three sets each proportional to each other:

x	20
y	50
30	150

Find x and y.

Solving using method A we can write:

$$\frac{x}{30} = \frac{20}{150} \text{ and } \frac{y}{30} = \frac{50}{150}$$

giving

$$x = \frac{600}{150} = 4 \text{ and } y = \frac{1500}{150} = 10$$

The fact that the vertical columns form two proportional sets could be used to give:

$$\frac{x}{20} = \frac{30}{150} \text{ and } \frac{y}{50} = \frac{30}{150}$$

leading to the same values of x and y.

The best approach in this case would be the use of the 'spotting' method C. The ratio of 150 to 30 is 5, so y is 50 divided by 5 = 10 and x is 20 divided by 5 = 4.

EXAMPLE 1.38

Find the values of a and b in the following proportional sets:

a	25	110
12	b	22

The best approach is by the 'spotting' method B. The ratio of 110 to 22 is 5, so a is 5 times 12 = 60 and b is 25 divided by 5 = 5.

EXAMPLE 1.39

Find the value of p in the two proportional sets:

36	9
22	p

The best approach is by the 'spotting' method C. The ratio of 36 to 9 is 4, so 22 is divided by 4 to give $p = 5.5$.

EXAMPLE 1.40

Find the values of x and y in the three proportional sets:

24	6
x	15
64	y

The best approach is by the 'spotting' method C. The ratio of 24 to 6 is 4, so x is 15 times 4 = 60 and y is 64 divided by 4 = 16.

EXAMPLE 1.41

Find the values of y and z in the two proportional sets:

y	18	21
9	z	63

The best approach is by the 'spotting' method B. The ratio of 63 to 21 is 3, so y is 9 divided by 3 = 3 and z is 18 times 3 = 54.

Note: From this point we will refer to methods B and C as the 'spotting' methods and to method A as the general method.

Setting up proportional sets for practical situations

We can now calculate missing values from two proportional sets of numbers, so let us now deal with the setting up of two proportional sets in solving practical examples.

For purposes of this general introduction, let us give the two proportional sets the titles set A and set B. Each of the numbers used in set A must be in the same units and the units should be stated after the title. The same situation must apply for numbers in set B.

We first need to identify the number that needs to be found and represent it by a letter. Then three known values need to be identified. One of them must be the value of the second set that corresponds to the required unknown value of the first set. The other two will be any known pair of values (one from each set) that correspond.

General situation:

set A (units for set A)   unknown value   known value

set B (units for set B)   known value   known value

Thus, for a particular situation, the form could be:

sodium chloride (mg)	x	450
water (mL)	12.5	50

Let us set up the proportional sets from the following example:

A suspension contains 120 mg of paracetamol in each 5 mL. Find the volume of suspension that contains 300 mg of paracetamol.

We said earlier: 'We first need to identify the number that needs to be found and represent it by a letter. Then three known values need to be identified. One of them must be the value of the second set that corresponds to the required unknown value of the first set. The other two will be any known pair of values (one from each set) that correspond.' Applying this to the example:

Let the volume of suspension required (mL) be x.

The amount of paracetamol that corresponds to this (in mg) is 300.

The known pair of corresponding values is made up of 5 mL and 120 mg.

Setting up the proportional sets:

volume of suspension (mL)	x	5
amount of paracetamol (mg)	300	120

We can now go on to solve for x.

EXAMPLE 1.42

The recommended dose of phenytoin for a patient is 840 mg. An injection contains 50 mg/mL. What volume of injection is needed for the recommended dose?

Let the required volume of injection (mL) be y. The corresponding known value is 840 mg and the known corresponding pair is made up of 1 mL and 50 mg. Setting up the proportional sets:

| amount of phenytoin (mg) | 840 | 50 |
| volume of injection (mL) | y | 1 |

We can then go on to solve for y.

EXAMPLE 1.43

1 L of aqueous solution contains 250 mL of syrup. How much syrup will be contained in 25 L of the solution?

Let the required amount of syrup in millilitres be x. Setting up proportional sets:

| volume of syrup (mL) | 250 | x |
| volume of solution (L) | 1 | 25 |

We can then go on to solve for x.

EXAMPLE 1.44

25 g of ointment contains 5 g of calamine. How much calamine will be contained in 60 g of ointment?

Let the required mass of calamine in grams be y. Setting up proportional sets:

| mass of calamine (g) | 5 | y |
| mass of ointment (g) | 25 | 60 |

We can then go on to solve for y.

Note: When the unknown value has been calculated it should be entered in the proportional sets table in place of the letter representing it and the user should then examine the table to check that the size of the calculated value seems to agree with corresponding values.

Proportional sets that become trivial

Consider the following example:

> *Calculate the number of tablets required for 7 days if 12 tablets are used each day.*

The reader will be able to give the number as 84, but note that the problem involves proportion and could be tackled as follows.

Let the required number of tablets be x. Setting up proportional sets:

number of tablets	12	x
number of days	1	7

We can 'spot' that 1 is multiplied by 12 to give 12, so 7 is multiplied by 12 to give $x = 84$. The number of tablets required is 84.

There is no virtue in going to the trouble of writing out proportional sets in cases such as this one, but it is useful to know that we are dealing with proportion.

Now consider the following example:

> *Find the volume of solution that contains 50 mg of a drug and has a concentration of 4 mg in 1 mL.*

Many readers will be able to give the volume as 12.5 mL, but this time some readers would probably welcome the help they would gain by writing down proportional sets.

Let the required volume of solution be y mL:

amount of drug (mg)	4	50
volume of solution (mL)	1	y

We can 'spot' that 4 is divided by 4 to give 1, so 50 is divided by 4 to give y:

$$y = \frac{50}{4} = 12.5$$

The volume of solution is 12.5 mL.

In tackling questions that involve a lot of information, it may be worth writing down proportional sets, including some that turn out to be rather trivial, in order to organise the information. The path to a solution will then probably become more obvious.

Practice calculations

Answers are given at the end of the chapter.

In questions 1 to 6 decide whether or not the pairs of sets are proportional.

Q1   6   8   10 . . .

         3   5   7 . . .

Q2   5   7   9 . . .

     20 28 36 . . .

Q3   2   3   4 . . .

     5   6   7 . . .

Q4   2   4   6 . . .

     5 10 15 . . .

Q5   25 35 . . .

      5   7 . . .

Q6   2   4   6 . . .

     3   6   9 . . .

Q7   Find the fraction that is equal to $\frac{7}{8}$ but has denominator 72.

Q8   Find the fraction that is equal to $\frac{4}{7}$ but has numerator 28.

Q9   Find the fraction that is equal to $\frac{2}{9}$ but has denominator 117.

Q10 Express $\frac{12}{20}$ in its lowest terms.

Q11 Express $\frac{3}{15}$ in its lowest terms.

Q12 Express $\frac{42}{54}$ in its lowest terms.

Q13 Express $\frac{78}{130}$ in its lowest terms.

Q14 Express $\frac{120}{42}$ in its lowest terms.

Q15 Multiply $\frac{3}{13}$ by 5.

Q16 Multiply $\frac{3}{17}$ by 4.

Q17 Multiply $\frac{5}{9}$ by 7.

Q18 Convert 0.8 to a fraction in its lowest terms.

Q19 Convert 0.87 to a fraction in its lowest terms.

Q20 Convert 0.875 to a fraction in its lowest terms.

Q21 Convert the fraction $\frac{5}{8}$ to a decimal.

Q22 Convert the fraction $\frac{7}{80}$ to a decimal.

Q23 Express 0.82 as a percentage.

Q24 Express 0.345 as a percentage.

Q25 Express 30% as a fraction in its lowest terms.

Q26 Express 0.3% as a fraction in its lowest terms.

Q27 Express $\frac{7}{8}$ as a percentage.

Q28 Express $\frac{6}{25}$ as a percentage.

Q29 Correct 213 471 to three significant figures.

Q30 Correct 213 871 to three significant figures.

Q31   Correct 213 571 to three significant figures.

Q32   Correct 0.004 221 to two significant figures.

Q33   Correct 0.004 252 to two significant figures.

Q34   Correct 2.5741 to two decimal places.

Q35   Correct 2.5755 to two decimal places.

Q36   Correct 1.7234 to three decimal places.

Q37   Correct 1.7236 to three decimal places.

Q38   Correct 1.7158 to two decimal places.

Questions 39 to 43 can be worked out using the 'spotting' methods.

Q39   Find the missing value x from the pair of proportional sets:

8   x 20

2   4   5

Q40   Find the missing number y from the pair of proportional sets:

25   30

y 6

Q41   Find the missing number z from the pair of proportional sets:

21   z

7   30

Q42   Find the missing number x from the pair of proportional sets:

81   18

x 2

Q43   Find the missing number y from the pair of proportional sets:

y 21

8   24

Q44   Find the missing number z from the pair of proportional sets:

4   10

10   z

Q45   Find the missing number x from the pair of proportional sets:

x 10

7   35

Q46   Find the missing number y from the pair of proportional sets:

32   y

19   41

Give your answer correct to two significant figures.

Q47   Find the missing number z from the pair of proportional sets:

225   420

192   z

Give your answer correct to three significant figures.

Q48   Find the missing number x from the pair of proportional sets:

x 11.3

22.5   15.7

Give your answer correct to three significant figures.

Answers

A1 Not proportional.

A2 Proportional. Each value of the lower set is four times the corresponding value of the upper set.

A3 Not proportional.

A4 Proportional. Each number of the lower set is 2.5 times the corresponding value of the upper set.

A5 Proportional. Each value of the upper set is five times the corresponding value of the lower set.

A6 Proportional. Each value of the lower set is 1.5 times the corresponding value of the upper set.

A7 $\frac{63}{72}$

A8 $\frac{28}{49}$

A9 $\frac{26}{117}$

A10 $\frac{3}{5}$

A11 $\frac{1}{5}$

A12 $\frac{7}{9}$

A13 $\frac{3}{5}$

A14 $\frac{20}{7} = 2\frac{6}{7}$

A15 $\frac{15}{13}$

A16 $\frac{12}{17}$

A17 $\frac{35}{9} = 3\frac{8}{9}$

A18 $\frac{4}{5}$

A19 $\frac{87}{100}$

A20 $\frac{7}{8}$

A21 0.625

A22 0.0875

A23 82%

A24 34.5%

A25 $\frac{3}{10}$

A26 $\frac{3}{1000}$

A27 87.5%

A28 24%

A29 213 000

A30 214 000

A31 214 000

A32 0.0042

A33 0.0043

A34 2.57

A35 2.58

A36 1.723

A37 1.724

A38 1.72

A39 16

A40 5

A41 90

A42 9

A43 7

A44 25

A45 2

A46 69

A47 358

A48 16.2

2

Systems of units

Mass and weight

Mass is the measure of quantity of matter. The Système International (SI) unit of mass is the kilogram (kg).

Weight is a force. The SI unit of force is the newton. A particle of mass 1 kg is attracted towards the centre of the earth by a force of g newtons, where g is the acceleration due to gravity and has a value that varies slightly at different points on the earth's surface. The value of g is about 9.8 m s^{-2}, so a mass of 1 kg has a weight of about 9.8 newtons.

In everyday life the word 'weight' is often used instead of the word 'mass'. A person's weight is stated as being, say, 160 kg and the units indicate that mass rather than force is implied. In pharmacy, 'weight' is traditionally used in cases where 'mass' would be more appropriate and where it is obvious from the context, and perhaps from the units, that a force is not intended. For example, tables of body weights are used, and in the *British Pharmacopoeia* (1999) concentration ratios are stated as being w/v or w/w, i.e. weight in volume and weight in weight. In each case it is mass rather than weight that is being considered.

Rather than always using the correct term 'mass' in this book, 'weight' is used to conform with current pharmacy texts. No forces are used, so whenever 'weight' occurs, 'mass' is implied.

Metric units

The units most commonly used in pharmacy are those of volume and mass. The basic metric unit of volume is the litre (L or l) and the basic metric unit of mass is the gram (g). (The litre is also the SI unit of volume, but the SI unit of mass is the kilogram (kg).)

Prefixes are used to indicate multiples and submultiples of units. Those in general use are shown in Table 2.1. Thus, for the basic unit of the litre, one thousand litres are equal to 1 kL and one thousandth of a litre is 1 mL. For the basic unit of the gram, one thousand grams are equal to 1 kg and one thousandth of a gram is 1 mg.

Table 2.1 Common prefixes

Prefix	mega	kilo	milli	micro
Factor	10^6	10^3	10^{-3}	10^{-6}
Symbol	M	k	m	μ

In this book the only units we use with prefixes are kg, mg, kL and mL. For other multiples or submultiples we write the word in full (e.g. microlitre, megagram).

The metric system is based on the decimal system (see p. 6) so, as with decimals, we have a system of 'place values'. Instead of column headings of units, hundreds, thousands, etc. we have:

Mass

megagrams – – kg – – g – – mg – – micrograms

Factors 10^6 10^5 10^4 10^3 10^2 10 1 10^{-1} 10^{-2} 10^{-3} 10^{-4} 10^{-5} 10^{-6}

Volume

megalitres – – kL – – L – – mL – – microlitres

There are other metric prefixes for some of the headings we have denoted by dashes, such as decigram and centigram, but we will not make use of them here.

Changing metric units

We can make use of 'place values' in changing metric units. Tackling the task in this way should avoid mistakes such as multiplying by a power of ten when division should have been carried out or vice versa.

EXAMPLE 2.1
_____

Change 200 mg to grams.

First write down column headings involving the relevant units, and underneath enter the 200 with the unit digit (the last zero) in the mg column. Fill the empty columns with zeros. The value in grams is read off by placing a decimal point after the digit in the grams column, i.e.

$$
\begin{array}{cccc}
\text{g} & - & - & \text{mg} \\
\end{array}
$$

200 mg = 0   2   0   0   = 0.2 g

EXAMPLE 2.2

Convert 5473 mL to litres.

$$
\begin{array}{cccc}
\text{L} & - & - & \text{mL} \\
\end{array}
$$

5473 mL = 5   4   7   3   = 5.473 L

EXAMPLE 2.3

Convert 1.26 mg to micrograms.

$$
\begin{array}{cccc}
\text{mg} & - & - & \text{micrograms} \\
\end{array}
$$

1.26 mg =   1   2   6   0   = 1260 micrograms

EXAMPLE 2.4

Convert 135465 micrograms to grams.

$$
\begin{array}{cccccc}
\text{g} & - & - & \text{mg} & - & - & \text{micrograms} \\
\end{array}
$$

135465 micrograms = 0   1   3   5   4   6   5   = 0.135465 g

EXAMPLE 2.5

Convert 0.003745 kL to mL.

$$
\begin{array}{cccccc}
\text{kL} & - & - & \text{L} & - & - & \text{mL} \\
\end{array}
$$

0.003745 kL =   0   0   0   3   7   4   5 = 3745 mL

Changing units between different systems of measurement

Units of measurement such as feet and inches, gallons and pints, and stones and pounds are still in everyday use. It may therefore be necessary to convert measurements between these systems and the metric system. Proportional sets can be used to aid the conversion. The relevant conversion factor must be found and used in the proportional sets, as in Example 2.6.

EXAMPLE 2.6
_____

Convert 3.4 pints to litres.

The conversion factor between the two sets of measurements is 1 L = 1.76 pints. Let the required number of litres be x. Setting up proportional sets:

litres	x	1
pints	3.4	1.76

Corresponding pairs are in the same ratio:

$$\frac{x}{3.4} = \frac{1}{1.76}$$

$$x = \frac{3.4}{1.76} = 1.93$$

3.4 pints = 1.93 L.

Note: Replacing the value for x in the proportional set allows us to check relative values and so to avoid errors.

....

Body-weight tables sometimes use weight in kilograms. Most people only know their weight in stones and pounds. It is therefore necessary to be able to convert values from one set of units to the other.

EXAMPLE 2.7
_____

Convert 106.4 kg to stones and pounds.

Conversion factor: 1 pound = 0.4536 kg.

Let the required number of pounds be y. Setting up proportional sets:

pounds	y	1
kilograms	106.4	0.4536

$$\frac{y}{106.4} = \frac{1}{0.4536}$$

$$y = \frac{106.4}{0.4536} = 234.56$$

106.4 kg is equal to 235 pounds (to the nearest pound). There are 14 pounds in 1 stone, so 235 pounds = 16 stone 11 pounds.

EXAMPLE 2.8

Convert 10 stone 4 pounds to kilograms.

Conversion factor: 1 pound = 0.4536 kg.

14 pounds = 1 stone, so 10 stone 4 pounds = 144 pounds.

Let the required number of kilograms be x. Setting up proportional sets:

pounds	1	144
kilograms	0.4536	x

Corresponding pairs are in the same ratio:

$$\frac{x}{144} = \frac{0.4536}{1}$$

$$x = 144 \times 0.4536 = 65.3$$

10 stone 14 pounds = 65.3 kg.

Conversions of temperature between degrees Fahrenheit and degrees Celsius

If we are given the information that 50 degrees Celsius = 122 degrees Fahrenheit, then to find the number of degrees Celsius (y) corresponding to 95 degrees Fahrenheit we may be tempted to set up sets of corresponding values:

degrees Celsius	50	y
degrees Fahrenheit	122	95

but beware: 75 degrees Celsius = 167 degrees Fahrenheit, so if we write sets of the two known corresponding pairs:

degrees Celsius	50	75
degrees Fahrenheit	122	167

we can see that the two sets are not proportional and therefore, we cannot equate ratios of corresponding pairs.

The freezing point of water is 0 degrees Celsius and 32 degrees Fahrenheit, so if we subtract 32 from Fahrenheit values we should then get a pair of proportional sets:

degrees Celsius	50	75
degrees Fahrenheit minus 32	90	135

90 = 50 times 1.8 and 135 = 75 times 1.8. The sets are proportional.

Returning to the task of finding the number of degrees Celsius (y) corresponding to 95 degrees Fahrenheit:

degrees Celsius	50	y
degrees Fahrenheit minus 32	122–32	95–32

Corresponding pairs are in the same ratio:

$$\frac{y}{63} = \frac{50}{90}$$

$$y = \frac{63 \times 50}{90} = 35$$

95 degrees Fahrenheit = 35 degrees Celsius.

Do not assume that all sets of corresponding values are proportional.

The boiling point of water on the Celsius scale is 100 degrees and on the Fahrenheit scale is 212 degrees, so the range of values between freezing point and boiling point is 100 degrees on the Celsius scale and 180 degrees on the Fahrenheit scale. It is therefore useful to use these ranges as corresponding values in changing values from one scale to the other.

EXAMPLE 2.9

Change 25 degrees Celsius to degrees Fahrenheit.

Let the corresponding number of degrees Fahrenheit be x. Setting up proportional sets:

degrees Fahrenheit minus 32	180	$x - 32$
degrees Celsius	100	25

Corresponding pairs are in the same ratio.
We can spot that 100 divided by 4 is 25, so 180 divided by 4 will be $x - 32$, therefore:

$$x - 32 = 45$$

$$x = 45 + 32 = 77$$

25 degrees Celsius = 77 degrees Fahrenheit.

EXAMPLE 2.10

Change 68 degrees Fahrenheit to degrees Celsius.

Let the required number of degrees Celsius be y. Setting up proportional sets:

degrees Fahrenheit minus 32	180	$68 - 32$
degrees Celsius	100	y

Corresponding pairs are in the same ratio:

$$\frac{y}{36} = \frac{100}{180}$$

$$y = \frac{100 \times 36}{180} = 20$$

68 degrees Fahrenheit = 20 degrees Celsius.

Practice calculations

Answers are given at the end of the chapter.

Q1   Change 0.035 g to milligrams.

Q2   Change 1384 mg to grams.

Q3   Change 437 mL to litres.

Q4   Change 12.47 L to millilitres.

Q5   Change 0.87 mL to microlitres.

Q6   Change 15750 microlitres to millilitres.

Q7   Change 0.0025 kg to grams.

Q8   Change 12 g to kilograms

Q9   Change 0.72 megalitres to kilolitres.

Q10   Change 145 kg to megagrams.

Q11   Use the conversion factor 1 L = 1.76 pints to express:
   (a)   6.43 pints in litres
   (b)   2.42 L in pints.

Q12   Use the conversion factor 1 pound = 0.4536 kg to express:
   (a)   9 stones 4 pounds in kilograms (1 stone = 14 pounds)
   (b)   49 kg in stones and pounds.

Q13   The boiling point of water is 100 degrees Celsius or 212 degrees Fahrenheit. The freezing point of water is 0 degrees Celsius or 32 degrees Fahrenheit. Express:
   (a)   15 degrees Celsius in degrees Fahrenheit (to the nearest degree)
   (b)   88 degrees Fahrenheit in degrees Celsius (to the nearest degree).

Answers

A1   35 mg

A2   1.384 g

A3   0.437 L

A4   12470 mL

A5   870 microlitres

A6   15.75 mL

A7   2.5 g

A8   0.012 kg

A9   720 kL

A10   0.145 megagrams

A11   (a)   3.65 L
         (b)   4.26 pints

A12   (a)   59 kg
         (b)   7 stone 10 pounds

A13   (a)   59 degrees Fahrenheit
         (b)   31 degrees Celsius

3

Concentrations

Introduction

Pharmaceutical preparations consist of a number of different ingredients in a vehicle to produce a product. The ingredients and vehicles used in a product can be solid, liquid or gas.

Concentration is an expression of the ratio of the amount of an ingredient to the amount of product. It can be expressed in several ways:

- in the case of a solid ingredient in a liquid vehicle the ratio is expressed as a weight in volume, denoted by w/v
- for a liquid ingredient in a solid vehicle the ratio is expressed as a volume in weight, denoted by v/w
- if both ingredient and vehicle are liquids the ratio is expressed as a volume in volume, denoted by v/v
- when the ingredient and vehicle are both solid the ratio is expressed as a weight in weight, denoted by w/w.

We know that rational numbers can be expressed as ratios, fractions, decimals or percentages. Since concentrations are expressions of ratios, they can also be expressed in different forms. The forms traditionally used are those of amount strengths, ratio strengths, parts per million and percentage strength. Each of these four forms can be expressions of w/w, v/v, w/v or v/w, depending on whether solids or liquids are involved.

For ratio strengths, parts per million and percentage strengths in w/w or v/v the amounts of ingredients and product must be expressed in the same units:

- a ratio of 7 mL to 12 mL is the ratio 7:12 v/v
- a ratio of 3 mg to 5 mg is the ratio 3:5 w/w.

As long as the units used are the same, they lead to the same ratio.

For a concentration of 3 mg to 5 g, we need to change to the same units before we can express the w/w ratio.

Converting 5 g to milligrams:

$$g \;\; - \;\; - \;\; mg$$

$$5\,g = \;\; 5 \;\; 0 \;\; 0 \;\; 0 \;\; = 5000\ mg$$

The ratio becomes 3 mg to 5000 mg, which is the ratio 3:5000 w/w.

In the case of w/v and v/w there is an agreed convention that states that weight is expressed in grams and volume is expressed in millilitres.

Let us now examine each of the traditional ways of expressing concentrations in more detail.

Amount strengths

Amount strengths can appear in any of the four forms, w/w, v/v, w/v or v/w. The amount strength is a ratio of the quantities and any units can be used, i.e. g/mL, mg/mL, mg/g, mL/mL, g/g, g/mL, etc. The units are stated in all cases.

Let us first consider a solid dissolved in a liquid to produce a solution.

EXAMPLE 3.1

A preparation contains 900 mg of sodium chloride dissolved in water to produce 100 mL of solution. Express the concentration of the solution as an amount strength.

The concentration of this solution can be expressed as an amount strength in units of mg/100 mL, mg/mL, g/100 mL, g/L and so on.

To convert the above concentration of sodium chloride solution into these different representations we use proportional sets. The solution contains the same concentration of sodium chloride irrespective of whether we have 100 mL, 50 mL or 1 mL. The ratio of sodium chloride to product is constant.

Let us consider how the concentration could be expressed as the ratio mg/mL and as the ratio g/mL.

Let the number of milligrams of sodium chloride in 1 mL of water be z. Setting up proportional sets:

sodium chloride (mg)	900	z
water (mL) to	100	1

The reason that we write *to* 100 mL rather than *in* 100 mL is that the sodium chloride is dissolved in water and made up to 100 mL with water. 900 mg of sodium chloride and 100 mL of water will produce more than 100 mL of solution therefore the amount of water required to make 100 mL of solution will be less than 100 mL because of the displacement caused by the sodium chloride. We will consider the concept of displacement and displacement values later. In addition, some drugs, such as strong concentrations of alcohol, may cause a contraction in volume when dissolved in water. For this reason, in Pharmacy we always make up *to* volume.

From the proportional sets, it can be spotted that $z = 9$, therefore the concentration of sodium chloride in this solution can be represented by an amount strength of 9 mg/mL.

Sodium chloride in water is a solid in a liquid and is therefore expressed as milligrams (a weight) in millilitres (a volume). This is a w/v ratio. We can also convert 9 mg to grams:

$$
\begin{array}{ccccc}
\text{g} & - & - & \text{mg} & \\
9 \text{ mg} = \quad 0 & 0 & 0 & 9 & = 0.009 \text{ g}
\end{array}
$$

The concentration of sodium chloride, which was earlier expressed as 9 mg/mL, can therefore also be represented by an amount strength of 0.009 g/mL.

Ratio strengths

Ratio strength is expressed as a ratio in the form 1 in r. The corresponding fraction would have a numerator of 1.

The agreed convention states that when ratio strength represents a solid in a liquid involving units of weight and volume then the weight is expressed in grams and the volume in millilitres.

1 in 500 potassium permanganate in water is a solid in a liquid and is therefore a weight in volume (w/v) ratio strength. This means that the solution contains 1 g of potassium permanganate made up to 500 mL with water.

EXAMPLE 3.2

---

2 L of an aqueous solution contains 200 mL of ethanol. Express this as a ratio strength.

Because this solution is a volume in volume we need to convert to the same units before we can express this as a ratio.
Converting 2 L into millilitres:

$$\begin{array}{ccccc} L & - & - & mL \\ 2\,L = & 2 & 0 & 0 & 0 & = 2000\text{ mL} \end{array}$$

Let the volume of product in millilitres containing 1 mL of ethanol be r. Setting up proportional sets:

ethanol (mL)   200   1

product (mL)   2000 r

By 'spotting', $r = 10$, therefore the ratio strength is 1 in 10 v/v.

....

Example 3.3 illustrates the calculation of a ratio strength for a solid in a solid.

EXAMPLE 3.3

---

5 g of product contains 250 mg of sulphur in yellow soft paraffin. Express this as a ratio strength.

This is a weight in weight product because both the sulphur and the yellow soft paraffin are solid. The weights must be converted to the same units before the concentration can be stated as a ratio strength.
Converting 250 mg to grams:

$$\begin{array}{ccccc} g & - & - & mg \\ 250\text{ mg} = & 0 & 2 & 5 & 0 & = 0.25\text{ g} \end{array}$$

Let the weight in grams of product containing 1 g of sulphur be r. Setting up proportional sets:

sulphur (g)   0.25   1

product (g)   5 r

Corresponding pairs are in the same ratio, therefore:

$$\frac{5}{0.25} = \frac{r}{1}$$

Solving for the unknown:

$$r = \frac{5}{0.25}$$

$$r = 20$$

The ratio strength is 1 in 20 w/w.

Parts per million

Parts per million (ppm) is used to denote concentrations in cases when the ratio of ingredient to product is very small. It is equivalent to a ratio in the form of p in 1 000 000 or a fraction in which the denominator is 1 000 000.

By the agreed convention, 1 ppm weight in volume is 1 g in 1 000 000 mL. 1 ppm weight in weight is 1 mg per 1 000 000 mg or 1 g per 1 000 000 g. In volume in volume it is 1 mL in 1 000 000 mL or 1 L in 1 000 000 L.

EXAMPLE 3.4

Fluoride in a water supply is expressed as parts per million w/v. Fluoride supplements should not be taken if the amount of fluoride in the water supply exceeds 0.7 parts per million w/v according to the British National Formulary (BNF). Express this ratio in mg/L.

By convention, 0.7 ppm can be represented as 0.7 g in 1 000 000 mL.
Converting 0.7 g to milligrams:

g   –   –   mg

0.7 g =   0   7   0   0   = 700 mg

Converting 1 000 000 mL into litres:

L   –   –   mL

1 000 000 mL = 1   0   0   0   0   0   0 = 1000 L

0.7 ppm w/v = 700 mg per 1000 L = 0.7 mg/L.

. . . .

EXAMPLE 3.5
_____

If the concentration of fluoride is 0.25 ppm w/v, how many litres would contain 1 mg of fluoride?

0.25 ppm w/v means 0.25 g per 1 000 000 mL.
    Converting 0.25 g to milligrams:

$$g \quad - \quad - \quad mg$$

0.25 g =   0   2   5   0   = 250 mg

Let the amount of product in millilitres containing 1 mg of fluoride be y. Setting up proportional sets:

fluoride (mg)   250   1

product (mL)   1 000 000 y

Corresponding pairs of values are in the same ratio so:

$$\frac{1000000}{250} = \frac{y}{1}$$

Solving for the unknown in the proportional sets:

$$y = \frac{1000000}{250}$$

$$y = 4000$$

Hence 4000 mL contains 1 mg of fluoride.
    Converting 4000 mL to litres:

$$L \quad - \quad - \quad mL$$

4000 mL =   4   0   0   0   = 4 L

4 L therefore contains 1 mg of fluoride.

. . . .

Percentage concentration

In terms of parts, a percentage is the amount of ingredient in 100 parts of the product. In the w/v and v/w cases, using the convention the units are grams per 100 mL and millilitres per 100 g.

EXAMPLE 3.6

Express 1 in 500 w/v solution of potassium permanganate as a percentage.

Let the number of grams of potassium permanganate in 100 mL of product be x. Setting up proportional sets:

potassium permanganate (g)	1	x
product (mL)	500	100

We can spot that we divide 500 by 5 to get 100, so we divide 1 by 5 to get $\frac{1}{5}$, therefore $x = 0.2$ and the percentage of potassium permanganate is 0.2% w/v.

EXAMPLE 3.7

Express 900 mg of sodium chloride made up to 100 mL with water as a percentage.

To express the value as a percentage, we need to convert the number of milligrams in 100 mL to grams in 100 mL:

$$\begin{array}{cccccc} & g & - & - & mg & \\ 900 \text{ mg} = & 0 & 9 & 0 & 0 & = 0.9 \text{ g} \end{array}$$

There is 0.9 g of sodium chloride in 100 mL of solution. The percentage is 0.9% w/v.

Converting expressions of concentration from one form to another

Let us consider a general case. Let the amount of the ingredient be a and the amount of product be b. Let p be the amount in 100 parts (the percentage concentration), 1 in r be the ratio strength and m be the number of parts per million.

We can set up the following proportional sets:

	amount	percentage	ratio strength	ppm
ingredient	a	p	1	m
product	b	100	r	1 000 000

This table shows the relationship between the different expressions of concentration. By using the proportional sets of the known expression of concentration and the required expression of concentration, it is possible to convert from one expression to another.

EXAMPLE 3.8

A solution contains 20 mL of ethanol in 500 mL of product. Express the concentration as a ratio strength and as a percentage strength.

Let p be the percentage strength and let the ratio strength be 1 in r. Setting up proportional sets as above:

	volume	ratio	percentage
ethanol (mL)	20	1	p
product (mL)	500	r	100

Corresponding pairs of values are in the same ratio so:

$$\frac{500}{20} = \frac{r}{1}$$

Solving for the unknown in the proportional sets:

$$r = \frac{500}{20}$$

$$r = 25$$

By 'spotting' we can see that $p = \frac{20}{5} = 4$, therefore the mixture can be expressed as the ratio strength 1 in 25 v/v or as the percentage strength 4% v/v.

EXAMPLE 3.9

A solid ingredient mixed with a solid vehicle has a ratio strength of 1 in 40. Find the percentage strength and the amount strength expressed as grams per gram.

Let p represent the percentage strength and let a grams be the weight of ingredient in 1 g of product. Setting up proportional sets:

	amount	percentage	amount strength (g/g)
ingredient (g)	1	p	a
product (g)	40	100	1

Corresponding pairs of values are in the same ratio so:

$$\frac{1}{40} = \frac{p}{100}$$

Solving for the unknown in the proportional sets:

$$p = \frac{100}{40}$$

$$p = 2.5$$

Corresponding pairs of values are in the same ratio so:

$$\frac{1}{40} = \frac{a}{1}$$

Solving for the unknown in the proportional sets:

$$a = \frac{1}{40}$$

$$a = 0.025$$

The concentration of the mixture can be expressed as either 2.5% w/v or 0.025 g/g.

EXAMPLE 3.10

A solution contains a solid dissolved in a liquid. The ratio strength is 1 in 2000 w/v. What are the percentage strength and the amount concentration expressed as mg/mL?

By convention, a ratio strength 1:2000 w/v means 1 g in 2000 mL, and the percentage strength is the number of grams of ingredient in 100 mL of product.

Let the percentage strength be p and the amount of solid in grams in 1 mL of product be a. Setting up proportional sets:

	ratio	*percentage*	*amount strength (g/mL)*
solid (g)	1	p	a
product (mL)	2000	100	1

Corresponding pairs of values are in the same ratio so:

$$\frac{1}{2000} = \frac{p}{100}$$

Solving for the unknown in the proportional sets:

$$p = \frac{100}{2000}$$

$$p = 0.05$$

Corresponding pairs of values are in the same ratio so:

$$\frac{1}{2000} = \frac{a}{1}$$

Solving for the unknown in the proportional sets:

$$a = \frac{1}{2000}$$

$$a = 0.0005 \text{ g}$$

Converting 0.0005 g to milligrams:

$$g \quad - \quad - \quad mg$$

$$0.0005 \text{ g} = \quad 0 \quad 0 \quad 0 \quad 0 \quad 5 = 0.5 \text{ mg}$$

The concentration of 1 in 2000 w/v can be expressed as 0.05% w/v or 0.5 mg/mL.

EXAMPLE 3.11

A liquid ingredient mixed with another liquid vehicle has a concentration of 5% v/v. Find the ratio strength and the amount strength expressed as mL/mL.

5% v/v can be expressed as 5 mL of ingredient in 100 mL of product.
    Let the ratio strength be 1 in r and the amount of ingredient in millilitres in 1 mL of product be a. Setting up proportional sets:

	percentage	*ratio*	*amount strength (mL/mL)*
ingredient (mL)	5	1	a
product (mL)	100	r	1

By 'spotting' we can see that:

$$r = \frac{100}{5} = 20$$

$$a = \frac{5}{100} = 0.05$$

The ratio is 1 in 20 v/v and the amount strength in mL/mL is 0.05 mL/mL.

EXAMPLE 3.12

5 g of solid ingredient is added to 45 g of a base. Find the percentage strength, the ratio strength and the amount strength expressed as g/g.

Remember that for weight in weight and volume in volume the product is equal to the sum of the vehicle and the ingredient, in this case 5 + 45 = 50 g.
    Let p be the percentage strength, 1 in r be the ratio strength and a grams be the amount in 1 g of product. Setting up proportional sets:

	amount	*percentage*	*ratio*	*amount strength (g/g)*
ingredient (g)	5	p	1	a
product (g)	50	100	r	1

By 'spotting' we can see that:

$$p = \left(5 \times \frac{100}{50}\right) = 10$$

$$r = \left(50 \times \frac{1}{5}\right) = 10$$

$$a = \left(5 \times \frac{1}{50}\right) = 0.1$$

The concentration can therefore be expressed as 10% w/w or 1 in 10 w/w or 0.1 g/g.

Calculating the amount of ingredient required to make up a percentage solution

In the same way as converting from one expression of concentration to another, it is also possible to use the proportional sets to calculate the amount of ingredient required to produce a known amount of a known percentage product.

This can be achieved by using the following proportional sets:

	amount	percentage
ingredient	a	p
product	b	100

Values p and b will be known and, therefore, a can be calculated.

EXAMPLE 3.13

How many milligrams of aluminium acetate are required to prepare 500 mL of a 0.03% w/v solution?

Aluminium acetate is a solid and is expressed as a weight, in this case milligrams. The vehicle is a liquid and is expressed in millilitres. By convention 0.03% w/v means 0.03 g in 100 mL therefore each 100 mL contains 0.03 g of aluminium acetate.

Converting 0.03 g to milligrams:

$$
\begin{array}{ccccc}
 & g & - & - & mg \\
0.03\ g = & 0 & 0 & 3\ 0 & = 30\ mg
\end{array}
$$

Let x be the number of milligrams of aluminium acetate in 500 mL. Setting up proportional sets:

aluminium acetate (mg)	x	30
product (mL)	500	100

By 'spotting' it can be seen that:

$$x = 30 \times 5 = 150$$

150 mg of aluminium acetate is required to produce 500 mL of a 0.03% w/v solution.

Calculating the amount of ingredient required to prepare a ratio strength solution

When the final concentration of the product is expressed as a ratio strength, then the following proportional sets can be used to calculate the amount of ingredient to produce a known amount of product.

	amount	ratio
ingredient	a	1
product	b	r

In this situation, r and b will be known and a will be calculated.

EXAMPLE 3.14

What is the amount of potassium permanganate in 300 mL of a 1 in 25 solution and what is the percentage strength of the solution?

By convention, a ratio strength of 1 in 25 means 1 g in 25 mL. Let a be the number of grams of potassium permanganate in

300 mL and p be the percentage strength. Setting up proportional sets:

	ratio	amount in 300 mL	percentage
potassium permanganate (g)	1	a	p
product (mL)	25	300	100

Corresponding pairs are in the same ratio:

$$\frac{a}{300} = \frac{1}{25}$$

Solving for the unknown:

$$a = \frac{1 \times 300}{25} = 12$$

Amount of potassium permanganate = 12 g.
By 'spotting' we can see that:

$$p = 1 \times 4 = 4$$

The solution therefore contains 4 g potassium permanganate in 100 mL = 4% w/v.
There are 12 g of potassium permanganate in 300 mL of solution and the percentage strength is 4% w/v.

....

Practice calculations

Answers are given at the end of the chapter.

Q1 Convert the following ratio strengths into percentage strengths:

(a) 1 in 25

(b) 1 in 20

(c) 1 in 50

(d) 1 in 800

(e) 1 in 500

(f) 1 in 2000

(g) 1 in 300

Q2   What is the concentration of the solutions, expressed as percentage strength and ratio strength, when the following amounts of drug Z are dissolved in enough water to produce 125 mL of solution?

(a) 25 g

(b) 50 g

(c) 60 g

(d) 5 g

(e) 7 g

Q3   If the following amounts of drug are made up to 5 g with lactose what is the percentage concentration of the resulting mix?

(a) 100 mg

(b) 150 mg

(c) 200 mg

(d) 300 mg

(e) 500 mg

Q4   How many milligrams of y are needed to make 200 mL of a 1 in 500 solution?

Q5   How many millilitres of y are needed to produce 400 mL of a 1 in 200 solution?

Q6   How many milligrams of y are needed to produce 25 g of a 1 in 5 ointment?

Q7   How many grams of y are there in 250 mL of a 1 in 80 solution?

Q8   Potassium permanganate   0.1 g

Purified water to   100 mL

How many millilitres of a 2.5% potassium permanganate solution could be used in place of the 0.1 g in the above formula?

Q9   How many milligrams of x are needed to make 5 mL of an 8% solution?

Q10   How many millilitres of x are needed to make 600 mL of a 3% solution?

Q11   How many milligrams of x are needed to make 200 mL of a 3.4% solution?

Q12   How many milligrams of x are there in 100 mL of a 0.01% solution?

Q13   How much calamine is required to produce 250 g of a 3% ointment?

Q14   What volume of 17% w/v solution contains 1.5 g of ingredient?

Q15   What volume of 20% w/v solution contains 5 g of ingredient?

Q16   What volume of 15% w/v solution contains 7 g of ingredient?

Q17   What volume of 34% w/v solution contains 150 g of ingredient?

Answers

A1   (a) 4%

      (b) 5%

      (c) 2%

      (d) 0.125%

      (e) 0.2%

      (f) 0.05%

      (g) 0.33%

A2   (a) 20%, 1 in 5

      (b) 40%, 1 in 2.5

      (c) 48%, 1 in 2.1

(d) 4%, 1 in 25
(e) 5.6%, 1 in 17.9

A3   (a) 2%
(b) 3%
(c) 4%
(d) 6%
(e) 10%

A4   400 mg

A5   2 mL

A6   5000 mg

A7   3.1 g

A8   4 mL

A9   400 mg

A10   18 mL

A11   6800 mg

A12   10 mg

A13   7.5 g

A14   8.8 mL

A15   25 mL

A16   46.7 mL

A17   441.2 mL

4

Dilutions

Simple dilutions

When a product is diluted there is a change in the amount of product, while at the same time the amount of ingredient in the product remains the same.

If a solution containing 5 g of an ingredient in 200 mL of product is diluted to 400 mL with vehicle, the final product becomes 400 mL, containing 5 g of ingredient. The volume of product has changed (it has doubled) and the amount of ingredient is still 5 g. The amount strength has therefore changed from 5 g/200 mL to 5 g/400 mL.

EXAMPLE 4.1

A product consists of a solid ingredient in a solid vehicle. 2 g of the solid ingredient is contained in 500 g of product. A further 250 g of vehicle is added to the product. Find the concentration of the diluted mixture as a percentage strength, a ratio strength and an amount strength in mg/g.

The amount of the ingredient will remain the same, i.e. 2 g. The total amount of product will change to 750 g:

	amount	_percentage_	_ratio_	_amount strength (g/g)_
ingredient (g)	2	p	1	a
product (g)	750	100	r	1

By setting up proportional sets and solving equations, or by 'spotting', we get:

$p = 0.27$

$r = 375$

$a = 0.0027$

Converting 0.0027 g to milligrams:

$$
\begin{array}{ccccccc}
 & \text{g} & - & - & & \text{mg} & \\
0.0027 \text{ g} = & 0 & 0 & 0 & 2 & 7 & = 2.7 \text{ mg}
\end{array}
$$

The diluted product has a percentage strength of 0.27% w/w, a ratio strength of 1 in 375 w/w and an amount strength of 2.7 mg/g.

....

Example 4.2 shows the method of calculating the final concentration of the diluted product starting with a ratio strength.

EXAMPLE 4.2

_____

100 mL of a 1 in 50 w/v solution is diluted to 1000 mL. Find the concentration of the diluted product as a percentage strength, a ratio strength and an amount strength expressed as mg/mL.

By convention, 1 in 50 means 1 g in 50 mL.
    Let the number of grams of ingredient in 100 mL of product be g. Setting up proportional sets:

  ingredient (g)   1 g
  product (mL)   50   100

By 'spotting':

  $g = 2$

therefore 100 mL of product contains 2 g of ingredient.
    After dilution, the amount of the ingredient remains the same (2 g) and the total amount of the vehicle becomes 1000 mL.
    Setting up proportional sets for the diluted product:

	amount	percentage	ratio	amount strength (g/mL)
ingredient (g)	2	p	1	a
product (mL)	1000	100	r	1

By 'spotting':

$p = 0.2$

$r = \left(\dfrac{1000}{2}\right) = 500$

$a = 0.002$

Converting 0.002 g to milligrams:

$$g \quad - \quad - \quad mg$$

0.002 g = 0 0 0 2 = 2 mg

The final solution can therefore be expressed as a percentage strength of 0.2% w/v or a ratio strength of 1 in 500 w/v or an amount strength of 2 mg/mL.

....

Serial dilutions

Rather than keeping large amounts of products in the dispensary it is usual to keep concentrated products. These stock solutions can then be diluted to the desired concentration for the final product.

Example 4.3 starts with a ratio strength.

EXAMPLE 4.3

_____

What volume of a 1 in 400 v/v solution is needed to produce 5 L of a 1 in 2000 v/v solution?

Let *y* mL be the volume of 1 in 400 solution required.

The amount of the ingredient is the same in both *y* mL of 1 in 400 solution and 5 L of 1 in 2000 solution. Let this amount be *x* mL. Setting up proportional sets:

for 1 in 400 v/v:

ingredient (mL)	1	*x*
product (mL)	400	*y*

for 5 L of 1 in 2000 v/v:

ingredient (mL)	1	x
product (mL)	2000	5000

From the second pair, by 'spotting':

$$x = \frac{5000}{2000} = 2.5$$

Now putting x in the first pair of proportional sets:

for 1 in 400 v/v:

ingredient (mL)	1	2.5
product (mL)	400	y

therefore

$$y = 400 \times 2.5 = 1000$$

so 1000 mL or 1 L of the 1 in 400 mixture is diluted to 5 L to produce a 1 in 2000 product.

....

Example 4.4 starts with a percentage strength.

EXAMPLE 4.4
_____

What volume of a 40% v/v solution needs to be used to produce 500 mL of 5% v/v solution?

Let y mL equal the volume of the 40% v/v solution required and let x mL equal the volume of ingredient in y mL of 40% v/v solution. There will also be x mL of ingredient in 500 mL of the 5% v/v solution. Setting up proportional sets:

for 40% v/v:

ingredient (mL)	40	x
product (mL)	100	y

for 500 mL of 5% v/v:

    ingredient (mL)   5 x

    product (mL)   100   500

By 'spotting':

    $x = 25$

Putting x in the first pair of proportional sets:

    for 40% v/v:

    ingredient (mL)   40   25

    product (mL)   100 y

Setting up and solving equations:

$$\frac{y}{25} = \frac{100}{40}$$

$$y = \frac{100 \times 25}{40}$$

$$y = 62.5$$

therefore 62.5 mL of the 40% v/v solution is required to produce 500 mL of 5% v/v solution.

....

Sometimes we are required to calculate the amount of diluent required to produce a stated final concentration.

EXAMPLE 4.5

To what volume must 250 mL of a 25% w/v solution be diluted to produce a 10% solution?

First calculate the amount of ingredient in 250 mL of 25% solution.

Let the number of grams of ingredient in 250 mL of 25% w/v solution be x. By convention, 25% w/v solution has 25 g of ingredient in 100 mL of product. Setting up proportional sets:

for 250 mL of a 25% w/v:

ingredient (g)   25 x

product (mL)   100   250

Corresponding pairs are in the same ratio:

$$\frac{25}{100} = \frac{x}{250}$$

Solving for the unknown value:

$$x = \frac{25 \times 250}{100}$$

$$x = 62.5$$

After dilution, the amount of the ingredient will stay the same, i.e. 62.5 g.
Let y mL be the final volume of the 10% w/v solution. Setting up proportional sets:

for 10% w/v:

ingredient (g)   10   62.5

product (mL)   100 y

By 'spotting' it can be seen that:

$$y = 625 \text{ mL}$$

We need to dilute 250 mL of a 25% w/v solution to 625 mL to produce a 10% w/v solution.

Concentrated waters

Concentrated waters, such as rose water, peppermint water and chloroform water, are used to produce single-strength products. They are used for dilution in the ratio 1 part of concentrated water with 39 parts of water. To produce the single-strength product, we take one part of the concentrate and dilute it to 40 parts with water.

Suppose that we have to make volumes of single-strength chloroform water (50 mL, 100 mL, 200 mL, 300 mL, 500 mL) from chloroform water concentrate. Since chloroform water concentrate is in the ratio 1: 40, we have to take 1 mL and dilute it to 40 mL with water in order to obtain single-strength chloroform water.

Setting up proportional sets:

chloroform water concentrate (mL)	1	a	b	c	d	e
water (mL) to		40	50	100	200	300	500

If we calculate the value for c:

$$\frac{1}{40} = \frac{c}{200}$$

$$c = \frac{200}{40} = 5$$

We therefore require 5 mL of chloroform water concentrate made up to 200 mL with water to produce 200 mL of single-strength chloroform water.

This calculation can be repeated for a, b, d and e. Alternatively, these values can be obtained from the value for c by 'spotting', as follows:

$$b = \frac{c}{2} = 2.5$$

$$a = \frac{b}{2} = 1.25$$

$$d = b \times 3 = 7.5$$

$$e = b \times 5 = 12.5$$

Thus, the following proportional sets are obtained for single-strength chloroform water:

chloroform water concentrate (mL)	1	1.25	2.5	5	7.5	12.5
water (mL) to		40	50		100	200	300	500

In most formulae the chloroform water is expressed as double strength for half the total volume. To make double-strength chloroform water we have to take twice the volume of the chloroform water concentrate.

To produce double-strength chloroform water:

chloroform water concentrate (mL)	2	2.5	5	10	15	25
water (mL) to		40	50	100	200	300 500

Triturations

One of the problems when weighing ingredients for preparations is that amounts of less than 100 mg cannot be weighed with sufficient accuracy. We have to use trituration to get the required amount.

EXAMPLE 4.6

How would you prepare 100 mL of a preparation to the following formula?

hyoscine hydrobromide (micrograms)	*500*
chloroform water (mL) to	*5*

Let y be the number of micrograms of hyoscine hydrobromide in 100 mL. Setting up proportional sets:

hyoscine hydrobromide (micrograms)	500	y
chloroform water (mL) to	5	100

By 'spotting':

y = 10000 micrograms

Converting 10000 micrograms to milligrams:

	mg	–	–	micrograms	
10000 micrograms =	1	0 0	0 0		= 10 mg

The problem we face is that we cannot weigh less than 100 mg with sufficient accuracy.

Let the number of millilitres of product that contains 100 mg of hyoscine hydrobromide be x. Setting up proportional sets:

hyoscine hydrobromide (mg)	10	100
chloroform water (mL) to	100	x

By 'spotting':

$x = 1000$

If we can only weigh 100 mg of hyoscine hydrobromide we would have to make this up to 1000 mL with chloroform water to get the required strength.

Alternative method

We could dissolve 100 mg of hyoscine hydrobromide in a known quantity of chloroform water (say 10 mL) and take out a volume of chloroform water that contained 10 mg of hyoscine hydrobromide and dilute this to 100 mL.

Let us weigh 100 mg of hyoscine hydrobromide and make up to 10 mL with chloroform water. We now need to know the number of millilitres of product that contains 10 mg of hyoscine hydrobromide. Let this be z. Setting up proportional sets:

hyoscine hydrobromide (mg)	100	10
chloroform water (mL) to	10	z

By 'spotting':

$z = 1$

If we take 1 mL of this solution we have 10 mg of hyoscine hydrobromide. We can then dilute this to 100 mL with chloroform water to get the required solution.

In the original method we used 1000 mL of chloroform water but in the alternative method only 110 mL was used.

If we had chosen to dissolve the 100 mg of hyoscine hydrobromide in 100 mL of chloroform water, we would proceed as follows.

Let a be the number of millilitres of product containing 10 mg of hyoscine hydrobromide. Setting up proportional sets:

hyoscine hydrobromide (mg)	100	10
chloroform water (mL) to	100	a

By 'spotting':

$$a = 10$$

We would make 10 mL of this solution up to 100 mL with chloroform water. In this situation we would use 200 mL of chloroform water overall.

The aim should be to dissolve the hyoscine hydrobromide to produce the required amount of solution with the least wastage. The solubility of the ingredient needs to be considered.

Powder calculations

The *Pharmaceutical Codex* states that powders must weigh a minimum of 120 mg. No maximum weight is stated. If the amount of drug in the powder is less than 120 mg, it is necessary to include an inert powder to bulk up the powder to the minimum weight.

EXAMPLE 4.7

Prepare five powders each containing 100 mg of paracetamol.

Setting up proportional sets for one and five powders:

number of powders	1	5
paracetamol (mg)	100	a
diluent (mg)	y	b
total weight (mg)	120	c

y is the amount of diluent required to increase the final weight of one powder to 120 mg, therefore:

$$y = 120 - 100 = 20$$

a is the amount of paracetamol in five powders, b is the amount of diluent and c is the total weight of the five powders. The ratio of the powders is 1 to 5 so we can calculate these values by multiplying by 5:

number of powders	1	5
paracetamol (mg)	100	500
diluent (mg)	20	100
total weight (mg)	120	600

To prepare five powders each containing 100 mg of paracetamol, we need to weigh 500 mg of paracetamol and add it to 100 mg of diluent. This mixture would then be divided into five powders of 120 mg.

In Example 4.8 powders containing a smaller quantity of drug are considered.

EXAMPLE 4.8

Prepare five powders each containing 10 mg of hyoscine hydrobromide.

Setting up proportional sets for one and five powders:

number of powders	1	5
hyoscine hydrobromide (mg)	10	a
diluent (mg)	y	b
total weight (mg)	120	c

therefore

$y = 120 - 10 = 110$

number of powders	1	5
hyoscine hydrobromide (mg)	10	50
diluent (mg)	110	550
total weight (mg)	120	600

As has been stated before we cannot accurately weigh less than 100 mg, so we have two alternatives: either make up the powders with 100 mg hyoscine hydrobromide or triturate the powders.

If we make up the powders with 100 mg of hyoscine hydrobromide we get:

number of powders	1	g
hyoscine hydrobromide (mg)	10	100
diluent (mg)	110	e
total weight (mg)	120	f

We can see that the hyoscine hydrobromide is in the ratio 1 to 10, therefore g, e and f are 10, 1100 and 1200, respectively, and we have therefore made enough for 10 powders.

Alternatively, we can use the trituration method. We take 100 mg of hyoscine hydrobromide and dilute it with 900 mg of diluent. We need to know what weight of powder contains 50 mg of hyoscine hydrobromide. Let that be n. Setting up proportional sets:

hyoscine hydrobromide (mg)	100	50
diluent (mg)	900	m
powder (mg)	1000	n

By 'spotting':

$n = 500$

We can therefore take 500 mg of this mixture and subtract that from the weight of five powders of 120 mg each:

$5 \times 120 = 600$ mg

Subtracting:

$600 - 500 = 100$ mg

If we take 500 mg of the triturate and add another 100 mg of diluent we have enough to make five powders each weighing 120 mg and containing 10 mg of hyoscine hydrobromide.

To prepare five powders of 10 mg hyoscine hydrobromide, we weigh 100 mg of hyoscine hydrobromide and add 900 mg of diluent. We then take 500 mg of this mixture and add 100 mg of diluent. The final mixture is then divided into five powders of 120 mg.

....

Example 4.9 shows how additional triturations can be used to achieve the required dose in the final product.

EXAMPLE 4.9

_____

Prepare six powders each containing 0.5 mg of drug.

Setting up proportional sets for one and six powders:

number of powders	1	6
drug (mg)	0.5	a
diluent (mg)	y	b
total weight (mg)	120	c

therefore:

$$y = 120 - 0.5 = 119.5$$

The figures are in the ratio of 1 to 6 so the proportional sets become:

number of powders	1	6
drug (mg)	0.5	3
diluent (mg)	119.5	717
total weight (mg)	120	720

Again we cannot weigh less than 100 mg of drug.
Let z equal the number of powders containing a total of 100 mg of drug:

number of powders	1	z
drug (mg)	0.5	100
diluent (mg)	119.5	d
total weight (mg)	120	e

By 'spotting':

$z = 200$

giving values for d and e:

number of powders	1	200
drug (mg)	0.5	100
diluent (mg)	119.5	23900
total weight (mg)	120	24000

We would have to make enough for 200 powders and try to mix 100 mg of drug with 23 900 mg of diluent.

Alternatively, we could use trituration. Weigh 100 mg of drug and mix with 900 mg and call this T1.

Let the weight of powder containing 3 mg of drug (i.e. sufficient for six powders) be y:

T1

drug (mg)	100	3
total weight (mg)	1000	y

By 'spotting'

$y = 30$

therefore 30 mg of powder contains 3 mg of drug.

We still cannot weigh this amount of powder, therefore we need to take 100 mg of T1 (which is 1/10th of the total product of T1, and will contain 10 mg of drug) and add 900 mg of diluent to produce T2.

Let the weight of T2 containing 3 mg of drug be z:

T2

drug (mg)	10	3
total weight (mg)	1000	z

In this case $z = 300$, therefore 300 mg of T2 contains 3 mg of drug, and we can weigh 300 mg.

The final weight for six powders is:

$6 \times 120 = 720$ mg

We therefore take 300 mg of T2 and subtract:

$720 - 300 = 420$ mg of diluent

By using this method we are creating different concentrations of mixtures:

T1 contains 100 mg of drug in 1000 mg of powder = 1 mg in 10 mg

T2 contains 10 mg of drug in 1000 mg of powder = 1 mg in 100 mg

T3 contains 1 mg of drug in 1000 mg of powder = 1 mg in 1000 mg etc.

Multiple dilutions

We now consider how to calculate the amount of ingredient required in the initial product when given the final concentration and the degree of dilution.

EXAMPLE 4.10

What weight of ingredient is required to produce 1000 mL of a solution such that when 2.5 mL of it is diluted to 50 mL with water it gives a 0.25% w/v solution?

Consider the 0.25% w/v solution and let y g be the weight of ingredient in 100 mL. By convention, 0.25% w/v means 0.25 g in 100 mL.

for 100 mL of 0.25% w/v:

ingredient (g)	0.25	y
water (mL) to	100	50

We can see that $y = 0.125$.

Now we take 2.5 mL of the original solution and increase the volume to 50 mL. The amount of ingredient will stay the same, i.e. y, therefore we get proportional sets that relate the weight of ingredient in 50 mL to the weight in 2.5 mL.

Let z be the number of grams of ingredient in 1000 mL of solution:

ingredient (g)	z	y
water (mL) to	1000	2.5

We know that $y = 0.125$, therefore:

ingredient (g)	z	0.125
water (mL) to	1000	2.5

By 'spotting':

$z = 50$

therefore the original solution is 50 g of ingredient made up to 1000 mL with water.

....

EXAMPLE 4.11
_____

What weight of malachite green oxalate is required to produce 500 mL of solution such that 25 mL of this solution diluted to 2000 L gives a 1 in 2 000 000 solution?

Start by converting the litres into millilitres so that all the units are the same:

$$L \; - \; - \; mL$$

2000 L =   2   0   0   0   0   0   0 = 2 000 000 mL

Let the amount of malachite green oxalate in 2 000 000 mL be y. Setting up proportional sets:

malachite green oxalate (g)	1	y
water (mL) to	2 000 000	2 000 000

By 'spotting':

$y = 1$

Since we took 25 mL of the original and diluted it to 2 000 000 mL, we know that 25 mL contains 1 g of malachite green oxalate because we have only increased the volume and the amount has stayed the same.

Let z be the amount of malachite green oxalate in the 500 mL of original solution. Setting up proportional sets:

malachite green oxalate (g)	z	1
water (mL) to	500	25

Corresponding values are in the same ratio:

$$\frac{z}{500} = \frac{1}{25}$$

Solving the equation for the unknown:

$$z = \frac{1 \times 500}{25} = 20$$

therefore 20 g of malachite green oxalate is dissolved in water to produce 500 mL of solution.

EXAMPLE 4.12

What weight of ingredient is required to produce 250 mL of a solution such that 10 mL of this solution diluted to 150 mL gives a 0.1% w/v solution?

Let z be the number of grams of ingredient in 250 mL of unknown strength product and y be the number of grams of ingredient in 10 mL of unknown strength product. The amount of ingredient in the final 150 mL of 0.1% solution will also be y. Setting up proportional sets:

for the unknown strength product:

ingredient (g) z y

product (mL)   250   10

for the final solution of 0.1% w/v:

ingredient (g) y 0.1

product (mL)   150   100

Corresponding values are in the same ratio:

$$\frac{y}{150} = \frac{0.1}{100}$$

Solving the equation for the unknown:

$$y = \frac{150 \times 0.1}{100}$$

$$y = 0.15$$

Putting this value into the first pair of proportional sets:

ingredient (g) z 0.15

product (mL)   250   10

Corresponding values are in the same ratio:

$$\frac{z}{250} = \frac{0.15}{10}$$

$$z = \frac{0.15 \times 250}{10} = 3.75$$

therefore we take 3.75 g of ingredient and make it up to 250 mL with water.

Examples 4.13 and 4.14 demonstrate how to calculate the amount of initial product of stated strength that is required to produce a stated volume of a final strength.

EXAMPLE 4.13
_____

How many millilitres of 0.5% w/v solution are required to produce 250 mL of 1 in 5000 solution?

By convention, 0.5% w/v means 0.5 g in 100 mL.

   Let the number of millilitres of 0.5% solution be y and let the number of grams of ingredient in 250 mL of a 1 in 5000 solution be x. The amount of ingredient in grams in y mL of 0.5% solution will also be x. Setting up proportional sets:

   for 0.5% w/v:

   ingredient (g)   0.5 x

   product (mL)   100 y

   for 250 mL of 1 in 5000:

   ingredient (g)   1 x

   product (mL)   5000   250

Corresponding pairs are in the same ratio:

$$\frac{1}{5000} = \frac{x}{250}$$

Solving for the unknown:

$$x = \frac{250}{5000}$$

$$x = 0.05$$

Substituting into the first pair of proportional sets:

   for 0.5% w/v:

   ingredient (g)   0.5   0.05

   product (mL)   100 y

By 'spotting':

$$y = 10$$

therefore 10 mL of 0.5% solution will produce 250 mL of 1 in 5000 solution.

....

EXAMPLE 4.14
_____

How many millilitres of a 1 in 80 w/v solution are required to make 500 mL of a 0.02% solution?

By convention, 1 in 80 means 1 g in 80 mL and 0.02% w/v means 0.02 g in 100 mL.

Let the number of millilitres of the 1in 80 solution be y and let the amount of ingredient in grams in 500 mL of 0.02% solution be x. The amount of ingredient in grams in y mL of 1 in 80 solution will also be x. Setting up proportional sets:

for 1 in 80:

ingredient (g)	1	x
product (mL)	80	y

for 500 mL of 0.02%:

ingredient (g)	0.02	x
product (mL)	100	500

By 'spotting':

$x = 0.1$

Substituting into the first pair of proportional sets:

for 1 in 80:

ingredient (g)	1	0.1
product (mL)	80	y

By 'spotting':

$y = 8$

therefore 8 mL of a 1 in 80 w/v solution is required to make 500 mL of a 0.02% w/v solution.

Mixing concentrations

There are situations when two or more strengths of product are mixed at stated volumes and the final concentration must be calculated.

EXAMPLE 4.15

What is the final % v/v of a solution if 200 mL of 40% v/v solution is added to 300 mL of 70% v/v solution?

The two volumes will be added together to make the final volume of 500 mL. The volumes of ingredients present in the two volumes will therefore need to be added together.

Let x mL be the volume of ingredient in 200 mL of 40% v/v solution. Setting up proportional sets:

ingredient (mL)	40	x
product (mL)	100	200

By 'spotting':

$x = 80$

Let y be the number of millilitres of ingredient in 300 mL of 70% v/v solution. Setting up proportional sets:

ingredient (mL)	70	y
product (mL)	100	300

By 'spotting':

$y = 210$

The total volume of ingredient in 500 mL of final solution is:

$80 + 210 = 290$ mL

Let p be the percentage strength. Setting up proportional sets:

ingredient (mL)   290 p

product (mL)   500   100

By 'spotting':

$p = 58$

therefore the final solution is 58% v/v.

....

Sometimes we are required to calculate the ratio in which two different products of given strengths must be mixed to produce a product of a given concentration.

Let us consider what happens when two products of different concentrations are mixed. The final volume is the sum of the two volumes and the final amount is the sum of the two amounts present in the volumes used.

For product 1 let the concentration be c_1, the volume of product used be v_1 and the amount of ingredient in v_1 be a_1. These values are c_2, v_2 and a_2 for product 2 and c_3, v_3 and a_3 for the final combined product. The volume of product 1 (v_1) + volume of product 2 (v_2) = volume of final product (v_3), i.e.

$$v_1 + v_2 = v_3$$

The amount of ingredient in v_1 (a_1) + amount of ingredient in v_2 (a_2) = amount of ingredient in v_3 (a_3), i.e.

$$a_1 + a_2 = a_3$$

If c_1 is the concentration of product 1 (expressed as a fraction or a decimal):

$$c_1 = \frac{a_1}{v_1}$$

$$a_1 = v_1 c_1$$

$$a_1 + a_2 = a_3$$

$$(v_1 \times c_1) + (v_2 \times c_2) = (v_3 \times c_3)$$

$$(v_1 \times c_1) + (v_2 \times c_2) = (v_1 + v_2) \times c_3$$

$$(v_1 \times c_1) + (v_2 \times c_2) = (v_1 \times c_3) + (v_2 \times c_3)$$

$$(v_1 \times c_1) - (v_1 \times c_3) = (v_2 \times c_3) - (v_2 \times c_2)$$

$$v_1 \times (c_1 - c_3) = v_2 \times (c_3 - c_2)$$

therefore:

$$\frac{v_1}{v_2} = \frac{c_3 - c_2}{c_1 - c_3}$$

EXAMPLE 4.16

Melleril suspension comes as thioridazine 100 mg/5 mL and 25 mg/5 mL solutions, which can be mixed to produce intermediate doses. If we want to produce a product that contains thioridazine 75 mg/5 mL, what proportion of the two mixtures do we need?

$$c_1 = \frac{100\ mg}{5\ ml} = 20$$

$$c_2 = \frac{25\ mg}{5\ ml} = 5$$

$$c_3 = \frac{75\ mg}{5\ ml} = 15$$

$$\frac{v_1}{v_2} = \frac{c_3 - c_2}{c_1 - c_3}$$

$$\frac{v_1}{v_2} = \frac{15 - 5}{20 - 15} = \frac{10}{5} = \frac{2}{1}$$

We therefore need 2 parts 100 mg/5 mL solution and 1 part 25 mg/5 mL solution to produce a 75 mg/5 mL solution.

We can show that this works if we are required to make 300 mL of 75 mg/5 mL Melleril suspension. Using the above proportions we add 2 parts of Melleril suspension containing thioridazine 100 mg/5 mL solution, i.e. 200 mL (v_1), and 1 part of the 25 mg/5 mL suspension, i.e. 100 mL (v_2).

Let a_1 be the amount of thioridazine in milligrams in 200 mL of 100 mg/5 mL Melleril suspension. Setting up proportional sets:

thioridazine (mg)	100	a_1
product (mL)	5	200

By 'spotting':

$a_1 = 4000$

Let y be the number of milligrams of thioridazine in 100 mL of 25 mg/5 mL Melleril suspension. Setting up proportional sets:

thioridazine (mg)	25	a_2
product (mL)	5	100

By 'spotting':

$a_2 = 500$

The amount of thioridazine in 300 mL of final product is a_3:

$a_1 + a_2 = a_3 = 4500$

Let the final strength be y mg thioridazine in 5 mL. Setting up proportional sets:

thioridazine (mg)	4500	y
product (mL)	300	5

Corresponding values are in the same ratio:

$$\frac{4500}{300} = \frac{y}{5}$$

Solving for the unknown:

$$y = \frac{4500 \times 5}{300}$$

$y = 75$

therefore the solution is 75 mg/5 mL, as expected.

EXAMPLE 4.17

Find the proportions of the same two suspensions given in Example 4.16 that would be required to produce a 50 mg/5 mL suspension.

$$c_1 = 20$$

$$c_2 = 5$$

$$c_3 = 10$$

$$\frac{v_1}{v_2} = \frac{10 - 5}{20 - 10} = \frac{5}{10} = \frac{1}{2}$$

We therefore mix 1 part 100 mg/5 mL solution with 2 parts 25 mg/5 mL solution.

EXAMPLE 4.18

What proportions of 90% v/v and 50% v/v ethanol mixtures would produce a 70% v/v mixture? Assume no contraction.

$$c_1 = \frac{90}{100} = 0.9$$

$$c_2 = \frac{50}{100} = 0.5$$

$$c_3 = \frac{70}{100} = 0.7$$

Provided that all the terms have the same denominator this division can be omitted.

$$\frac{v_1}{v_2} = \frac{0.7 - 0.5}{0.9 - 0.7} = \frac{0.2}{0.2} = \frac{1}{1}$$

We therefore need to mix 1 part 90% solution with 1 part 50% solution.

We can prove this is correct. If we mix 100 mL of 90% solution and 100 mL of 50% solution we expect the final strength to be 70%.

Let a_1 be the number of millilitres of ethanol in 100 mL of 90% solution. Setting up proportional sets:

ethanol (mL)	90	a_1
product (mL)	100	100

By 'spotting':

$a_1 = 90$

Let a_2 be the number of millilitres of ethanol in 100 mL of 50% solution. Setting up proportional sets:

ethanol (mL)	50	a_2
product (mL)	100	100

By 'spotting':

$a_2 = 50$

therefore the final product contains an ethanol volume of a_3 in 200 mL.

$a_3 = a_1 + a_2 = 50 + 90 = 140$

Let p be the percentage strength of the final product. Setting up proportional sets:

ethanol (mL)	140	p
product (mL)	200	100

By 'spotting':

$p = 70$

therefore the final product is 70% v/v and the ratio is correct.

....

Practice calculations

Answers are given at the end of the chapter.

Q1   What weight of potassium permanganate is required to produce 300 mL of solution such that 5 mL of this solution diluted to 250 mL gives a 0.01% w/v solution?

Q2   What weight of potassium permanganate is required to produce 500 mL of solution such that 25 mL of this solution diluted to 500 mL gives a 0.025% w/v solution?

Q3   What weight of zinc sulphate is required to produce 150 mL of solution such that 10 mL of this solution diluted to 200 mL gives a 1% w/v solution?

Q4   What weight of potassium permanganate is required to produce 200 mL of solution such that 50 mL of this solution diluted to 200 mL will produce a 1 in 400 solution?

Q5   What weight of malachite green oxalate is required to produce 300 mL of a solution such that 25 mL of this solution diluted to 2000 L gives a 0.5 ppm solution?

Q6   How many millilitres of water must be added to 180 mL of 40% v/v solution in order to produce a 5% v/v solution?

Q7   What weight of copper sulphate is required to produce 150 mL of solution such that 30 mL of this solution diluted to 150 mL produces a 1 in 6000 solution?

Q8   What weight of potassium permanganate is needed to produce 300 mL of solution such that if 1 mL is diluted to 20 mL a 0.1% w/v solution is produced?

Q9   What volume of thioridazine 100 mg/5 mL is required to be diluted to give 200 mL of 75 mg/5 mL solution?

Q10   How many millilitres of 90% alcohol when diluted to 135 mL produces 60% alcohol? (Assume no contraction in volume)

Q11   When 70 mL of sodium chloride 0.9% w/v solution is combined with 100 mL of 1.7% w/v sodium chloride solution what is the final strength of the solution?

Q12   What volume of a 0.6% w/v solution is required to produce 200 mL of 1 in 10 000 solution?

Q13   What volume of a 1 in 50 solution is required to produce 300 mL of a 0.3% w/v solution?

Q14   Calculate the volumes of two stock solutions of 100 mg/5 mL and 25 mg/5 mL that must be mixed to produce 500 mL of 75 mg/5 mL solution.

Q15   What volumes of two stock solutions of 30% w/v and 60% w/v are required to make 300 mL of 40% w/v solution?

Q16   Calculate the volume of 0.2% w/v potassium permanganate solution required to produce 1000 mL of a 100 ppm solution.

Answers

A1   1.5 g

A2   2.5 g

A3   30 g

A4   2 g

A5   12 mg

A6   1260 mL

A7   125 mg

A8   6 g

A9   150 mL

A10   90 mL

A11   1.37%

A12   3.3 mL

A13   45 mL

A14   167 mL of 25 mg/5 mL solution and 333 mL of 100 mg/5 mL solution

A15   100 mL of 60% solution and 200 mL of 30% solution

A16   50 mL

5

Formulations

Formulae in pharmacy are recipes either from the standard literature available or from the directions of the prescriber. Ingredients can be listed as amounts, parts or percentages.

The formula may also have the amount in a greater or smaller quantity than is prescribed on the prescription. Formulae in the *British Pharmacopoeia* tend to make 1000 mL or 1000 g of product, whereas formulae in the BNF tend to make 10 mL or 10 g of product.

Since ingredients with a formula have to be kept in fixed ratios, they form proportional sets. Comparison of numbers in the sets after calculation to ensure that the proportions are maintained is a valuable way of checking the formula and should overcome the potential for error.

Using proportional sets provides a structured approach to the problem and provides you with a method for checking accuracy.

Reducing the formula

Some reference sources provide a formula for a larger quantity than the quantity required on the prescription.

EXAMPLE 5.1

A prescription requires 200 mL of Chalk Mixture, Paediatric BP. The formula is:

chalk	*20 g*
tragacanth powder	*2 g*
cinnamon water, concentrated	*4 mL*
syrup	*100 mL*
chloroform water, double strength	*500 mL*
water for preparation to	*1000 mL*

We therefore have a formula to produce 1000 mL of the preparation but require 200 mL. Calculate the quantities required to produce 200 mL.

Setting up proportional sets:

	master formula	to make 200 mL
chalk (g)	20	*a*
tragacanth powder (g)	2	*b*
cinnamon water, concentrated (mL)	4	*c*
syrup (mL)	100	*d*
chloroform water, double strength (mL)	500	*e*
water for preparation (mL) to	1000	200

We can calculate the missing values by setting up the ratio equations for corresponding pairs or by spotting.
To calculate the amount of chalk we pick out the proportional sets:

chalk (g)	20	*a*
water for preparation (mL) to	1000	200

By 'spotting', 1000 is divided by five to get 200, so 20 is divided by five to get:

$a = 4$

Continuing the process for other pairs of ingredients we get:

	master formula	to make 200 mL
chalk (g)	20	4
tragacanth powder (g)	2	0.4
cinnamon water, concentrated (mL)	4	0.8
syrup (mL)	100	20

chloroform water, double strength (mL)	500	100
water for preparation (mL) to	1000	200

At this stage it is important to check the relative amounts of the ingredients and re-check the ratios in order to eliminate any errors.

Increasing the formula

Some reference sources provide a formula that is for a smaller quantity than the quantity required on the prescription.

EXAMPLE 5.2

Calculate the quantities required to produce 300 mL of Aromatic Magnesium Carbonate Mixture BP using the formula:

light magnesium carbonate	*300 mg*
sodium bicarbonate	*500 mg*
aromatic cardamom tincture	*0.3 mL*
chloroform water, double strength	*5 mL*
water to	*10 mL*

Setting up proportional sets:

	master formula	to make 300 mL
light magnesium carbonate (mg)	300	a
sodium bicarbonate (mg)	500	b
aromatic cardamom tincture (mL)	0.3	c
chloroform water, double strength (mL)	5	d
water (mL) to	10	300

Picking out two proportional sets:

light magnesium carbonate (mg)	300	*a*
water (mL) to	10	300

Corresponding pairs are in the same ratio so:

$$\frac{300}{10} = \frac{a}{300}$$

Solving for the unknown:

$$a = \frac{300 \times 300}{10}$$

$$a = 9000$$

We continue the process to get:

	master formula	to make 300 mL
light magnesium carbonate (mg)	300	9000
sodium bicarbonate (mg)	500	15 000
aromatic cardamom tincture (mL)	0.3	9
chloroform water, double strength (mL)	5	150
water (mL) to	10	300

Again, a thorough check of the corresponding values should be made.

Formulae involving parts

Sometimes the formula for a product is expressed as parts rather than as quantities. The total amount of product will be the sum of the parts of the ingredients. From this, a formula can be produced and used to calculate the amounts of the ingredients in a required amount of product.

EXAMPLE 5.3

Consider the standard for Industrial Methylated Spirit (IMS) BP, which states that ingredients should be in the ratio 95 parts spirit to 5 parts wood naphtha. It is not uncommon for the ingredients to be expressed in a ratio of parts. In IMS both the ingredients are liquids therefore the parts are volume in volume. How much of each ingredient is required to produce 300 L?

Setting up proportional sets:

	master formula	to make 300 L
spirit (L)	95	a
wood naphtha (L)	5	b
IMS (L)	100 (95 + 5)	300

We can spot that:

$b = 5 \times 3 = 15$

$a = 95 \times 3 = 285$

therefore the proportional sets become:

	master formula	to make 300 L
spirit (L)	95	285
wood naphtha (L)	5	15
IMS (L)	100	300

Example 5.4 involves solids in a formula expressed as parts.

EXAMPLE 5.4

Find the quantities of ingredients needed to produce 50 g of product using the formula:

calamine (parts weight)   2

yellow soft paraffin (parts weight)   38

The total ointment contains 40 parts (2 + 38). Setting up the proportional sets:

	master formula	to produce 50 g
calamine (g)	2	x
yellow soft paraffin (g)	38	y
total (g)	40	50

Corresponding pairs of values are in the same ratio:

$$\frac{2}{40} = \frac{x}{50}$$

Solving for the unknown:

$$x = \frac{2 \times 50}{40}$$

$$x = 2.5$$

therefore:

$$y = 50 - 2.5 = 47.5$$

The proportional sets become:

	master formula	to produce 50 g
calamine (g)	2	2.5
yellow soft paraffin (g)	38	47.5
total (g)	40	50

It is necessary to differentiate carefully between the use of 'parts' and 'to parts'. Compare the following two formulae:

Formula 1

calamine	1 part
white soft paraffin	10 parts

This is equivalent to:

calamine	1 g
white soft paraffin	10 g

This is a total of 11 g (or 11 parts).

Formula 2

calamine	1 part
white soft paraffin to	10 parts

This is equivalent to:

calamine	1 g
white soft paraffin	9 g

This is a total of 10 g (or 10 parts).

Formulae containing percentages

A formula can also be expressed in percentages. Ointments and creams are the most common examples of this. The percentages of the ingredients can be used to produce the formula, and the ingredients in a known amount of product can be calculated.

EXAMPLE 5.5

Using the following formula, calculate the amounts of ingredients required to make 25 g:

sulphur	*6%*
salicylic acid	*4%*
white soft paraffin to	*100%*

Setting up proportional sets:

	master formula	to make 25 g
sulphur (g)	6	a
salicylic acid (g)	4	b
white soft paraffin (g)	90	c
total ointment (g)	100	25

100 is divided by four to get 25, therefore by 'spotting', each amount in the first column is divided by four to get the corresponding amount in the second column. The result is:

	master formula	to make 25 g
sulphur (g)	6	1.5
salicylic acid (g)	4	1
white soft paraffin (g)	90	22.5
total ointment (g)	100	25

EXAMPLE 5.6

Find the amount of ingredients required to make 50 g of the following formulation:

calamine	*6% w/w*
liquid paraffin	*7% w/w*
yellow soft paraffin to	*100% w/w*

Setting up proportional sets:

	master formula	to make 50 g
calamine (g)	6	a
liquid paraffin (g)	7	b

yellow soft paraffin (g)	87	c
total product	100	50

By 'spotting':

$a = 3$

$b = 3.5$

$c = 43.5$

The formula is therefore:

	master formula	*to make 50 g*
calamine (g)	6	3
liquid paraffin (g)	7	3.5
yellow soft paraffin (g)	87	43.5

Practice calculations

Answers are given at the end of the chapter.

Q1 Calculate the amounts of the following required to produce 200 g of cream:

calamine	10%
zinc oxide	15%
aqueous cream to	100%

Q2 Calculate the formula for 20 g of benzoic acid ointment compound using the formula:

benzoic acid	6%
salicylic acid	4%
(in emulsifying ointment)	

Q3 Calculate the formula required to produce 300 mL of menthol and eucalyptus inhalation from the formula:

menthol	2 g
eucalyptus oil	10 g
light magnesium carbonate	7 g
water to	100 mL

Q4 Calculate the amounts of ingredients required to make 30 g of ointment to the following formula:

coal tar solution	12% w/w
hydrous wool fat	24% w/w
yellow soft paraffin to	100%

Q5 Calamine and Coal Tar Ointment BP has the following formula:

calamine	12.5 g
strong coal tar solution	2.5 g
zinc oxide	12.5 g
hydrous wool fat	25 g
white soft paraffin	47.5 g

Calculate the amounts of ingredients required to produce 25 g of product.

Q6 Zinc and coal tar paste has the following formula:

zinc oxide	6% w/w
coal tar	6% w/w
emulsifying wax	5% w/w
starch	38% w/w
yellow soft paraffin	45% w/w

Calculate the amounts of ingredients required to produce 300 g of paste.

Q7 Calculate the amounts of ingredients required to produce 300 mL of Ammonia and Ipecacuanha Mixture BP, which has the formula:

ammonium bicarbonate	200 mg
liquorice liquid extract	0.5 mL
ipecacuanha tincture	0.3 mL

concentrated camphor water 0.1 mL
concentrated anise water 0.05 mL
double-strength chloroform water 5 mL
water to 10 mL

Q8 Calculate the amounts of ingredients required to make 150 mL of Diamorphine Linctus 1973, which has the formula:

diamorphine hydrochloride 3 mg
oxymel 1.25 mL
glycerol 1.25 mL
compound tartrazine solution 0.06 mL
syrup to 5 mL

Q9 Calculate the amounts of ingredients required to make 3 L of the formula:

witch hazel 4 parts
glycerol 1 part
water 15 parts

Q10 Calculate the amounts of ingredients required to make 2 L of the formula:

aluminium hydroxide 200 mg
activated dimethicone 25 mg
magnesium hydroxide 200 mg
water to 5 mL

Q11 Calculate the amounts of ingredients required to make 30 g of coal tar and zinc ointment using the formula:

strong coal tar solution 100 g
zinc oxide, finely sifted 300 g
yellow soft paraffin 600 g

Q12 Calculate the amounts of ingredients needed to produce 200 mL of kaolin and morphine mixture using the formula:

light kaolin 200 g
sodium bicarbonate 50 g
chloroform and morphine tincture 40 mL
water sufficient to produce 1000 mL

Q13 Calculate using the following formula the amounts of ingredients needed to produce 500 g of product:

calcium carbonate	5 parts
sodium bicarbonate	5 parts
bismuth subcarbonate	3 parts

Q14 Calculate the amounts of ingredients required to make 200 g of product from the formula:

Betnovate ointment	1 part
yellow soft paraffin to	5 parts

Q15 Calculate the amounts of ingredients required to make 300 g of product from the formula:

Betnovate ointment	3 parts
yellow soft paraffin	8 parts

Answers

A1
calamine	20 g
zinc oxide	30 g
aqueous cream	150 g

A2
benzoic acid	1.2 g
salicylic acid	0.8 g
emulsifying ointment	18 g

A3
menthol	6 g
eucalyptus oil	30 g
light magnesium carbonate	21 g
water to	300 mL

A4
coal tar solution	3.6 g
hydrous wool fat	7.2 g
yellow soft paraffin	19.2 g

A5
calamine	3.125 g
strong coal tar solution	0.625 g
zinc oxide	3.125 g
hydrous wool fat	6.25 g
white soft paraffin	11.875 g

A6   zinc oxide   18 g
    coal tar   18 g
    emulsifying wax   15 g
    starch   114 g
    yellow soft paraffin   135 g

A7   ammonium bicarbonate   6000 mg
    liquorice liquid extract   15 mL
    ipecacuanha tincture   9 mL
    concentrated camphor water   3 mL
    concentrated anise water   1.5 mL
    double-strength chloroform water   150 mL
    water to   300 mL

A8   diamorphine hydrochloride   90 mg
    oxymel   37.5 mL
    glycerol   37.5 mL
    compound tartrazine solution   1.8 mL
    syrup to   150 mL

A9   witch hazel   0.6 L
    glycerol   0.15 L
    water   2.25 L

A10   aluminium hydroxide   80 000 mg
    activated dimethicone 10 000 mg
    magnesium hydroxide   80 000 mg
    water to   2000 mL

A11   strong coal tar solution   3 g
    zinc oxide, finely sifted   9 g
    yellow soft paraffin   18 g

A12   light kaolin   40 g
    sodium bicarbonate   10 g
    chloroform and morphine tincture   8 mL
    water sufficient to produce   200 mL

A13   calcium carbonate   192.3 g
    sodium bicarbonate   192.3 g
    bismuth subcarbonate   115.4 g

A14   Betnovate ointment   40 g
         yellow soft paraffin   160 g

A15   Betnovate ointment   81.8 g
         yellow soft paraffin   218.2 g

6

Calculation of doses

Definition of dose and dosage regimen

A *dose* is the quantity or amount of a drug or drug formulation taken by, or administered to, a patient to achieve a therapeutic outcome.

The term 'dose' can be further qualified as a *single dose*, a *daily dose*, a *daily divided dose*, a *weekly dose* or a *total dose*, etc., as described below.

- **single dose:** for example, in the treatment of threadworm, the BNF recommended dose for mebendazole is expressed as 100 mg, i.e. a single dose of 100 mg
- **daily dose:** an example of a daily dose is the BNF recommended dose of digitoxin, which is stated as 100 micrograms daily
- **daily divided dose:** the recommended dose for doxepin is 75 mg daily in divided doses, i.e. the 75 mg dose is divided into smaller amounts such that a total of 75 mg is given per day
- **weekly dose:** chloroquine, when used as an antimalarial, has a dosage regimen of 250 mg once weekly
- **total dose:** treosulfan has a BNF recommended total dose range of 21–28 g.

The dose of a drug may be *repeated*. For example, in the case of mebendazole, the BNF states 'if re-infection [with threadworm] occurs a second dose may be needed after 2–3 weeks'.

Additionally, a dose may be repeated regularly either throughout the day or some other time period. Such scheduling of doses is called the *dosage regimen*. Examples of different dosage regimens are:

- in the treatment of whipworm, the BNF recommended dosage of mebendazole is 100 mg twice daily for 3 days, i.e. the dose is 100 mg of mebendazole and the dosage regimen is twice daily for 3 days
- ampicillin has a dosage regimen of 0.25–1.0 g to be taken orally every 6 hours
- metronidazole, when used in the oral treatment of leg ulcers, has a dosage regimen of 400 mg every 8 hours for 7 days.

Thus doses and dosage regimens vary with the drug and the disease/illness/symptoms that the drug is intended to treat. The dose and dosage regimen of a drug can be found in official publications, such as the BNF, and in manufacturers' literature.

In addition, a drug may be presented in more than one formulation and in more than one strength. For example, the drug carbamazepine is available in the following formulations:

tablets: 100 mg, 200 mg and 400 mg

liquid: 100 mg/5 mL

suppositories: 125 mg and 250 mg

A prescription stating the dose as 100 mg carbamazepine could mean that the prescriber wants a 100 mg tablet or 5 mL of the liquid. In such a situation the pharmacist would need to make a judgement or query the prescriber's intentions.

Doses based on units of formulations

Solid formulations

The doses of many formulations that contain more than one active ingredient are expressed as units of the dosage form. Examples of combinations of drugs are the compound analgesics:

co-codaprin (aspirin and codeine phosphate)

co-codamol (codeine phosphate and paracetamol)

co-proxamol (paracetamol and dextropropoxyphene hydrochloride)

and combinations of diuretics:

co-amilozide (amiloride hydrochloride and hydrochlorothiazide)

co-amilofruse (amiloride hydrochloride and furosemide (frusemide)).

Examples of units of solid dosage forms are tablets, capsules, sachets and suppositories. The doses of such pharmaceutical products are expressed as one or more units. These doses may be part of a dosage regimen, for example two tablets at night for 3 days.

The calculations involving such unit doses are relatively simple and are normally concerned with calculating a total number of dose units for a specific treatment period.

EXAMPLE 6.1

Calculate the total number of tablets to be dispensed if a prescription requires three tablets of drug X four times a day for 7 days.

Number of tablets per day is:

$3 \times 4 = 12$

Number of tablets for 7 days is:

$12 \times 7 = 84$

84 tablets should be dispensed.

Some prescribers specify the number of days of treatment by using abbreviations. For example:

- days may be expressed as a fraction of a week, thus 3 days will be represented as 3/7 and 5 days as 5/7
- weeks may be represented as a fraction of the number of weeks in the year, thus 2 weeks will be written as 2/52 and 6 weeks as 6/52
- months may be represented as a fraction of the number of months in a year, thus 6 months will be written as 6/12 and 9 months as 9/12.

If a prescriber uses such an abbreviation, the calculation of the total number of dose units follows the same method as above.

EXAMPLE 6.2

A prescription requires two sachets of drug Y four times a day for 3/7. How many sachets should be supplied?

Number of sachets per day = 8.
3/7 is the abbreviation for 3 days.

Total number of sachets is:

$$8 \times 3 = 24$$

24 sachets should be supplied.

Liquid formulations

The normal unit of measurement for oral liquid medicines is the 5 mL spoon or multiples thereof. Some medicinal products have a dose or dose range larger than 5 mL. For example, liquid paraffin emulsion has a dose range of 10–30 mL. Such a dose range will need to be converted into units of 5 mL, that is two to six 5 mL spoonfuls.

With doses of liquid medicines it is important not to confuse 5 mL doses with the total volume of medicine to be supplied.

EXAMPLE 6.3

A prescription requires a patient to receive a quantity of indigestion mixture with a dosage regimen of 20 mL three times a day for 5 days. Calculate the number of doses and the total volume supplied to the patient.

Total number of doses is:

$$3 \times 5 = 15$$

Total volume is:

$$15 \times 20 \text{ mL} = 300 \text{ mL}$$

The pharmacist needs to dispense 300 mL, which is a total of 15 doses.

In some situations it may be necessary to calculate the length of time taken to use up the total volume of medicine supplied. Such a situation is illustrated in Example 6.4.

EXAMPLE 6.4

A patient buys a 200 mL bottle of cough mixture. The dosage regimen is two 5 mL spoonfuls four times a day. If the patient takes the mixture according to the dosage regimen, for how many days will the mixture last?

The dosage regimen is two 5 mL spoonfuls (that is 10 mL) four times a day, therefore the total volume used per day is 40 mL. The total volume of mixture supplied to the patient is 200 mL, therefore the number of days the mixture will last for is:

$$\frac{200}{40} = 5$$

The mixture will be used up by the end of 5 days.

If the dose that would be contained in a 5 mL spoonful is too large for the patient, then doses smaller than 5 mL may be given using a 5 mL oral syringe. The 5 mL oral syringe is calibrated into 0.5 mL divisions from 1 to 5 mL. Thus, it is possible to deliver volumes between 1 and 5 mL using the oral syringe. The volumes delivered by the oral syringe are usually used for children or very frail adult patients. Example 6.5 demonstrates the calculation of the total volume to be dispensed when a dose volume of less than 5 mL is prescribed.

EXAMPLE 6.5

A very young child is prescribed 2.0 mL of a cough mixture three times a day for 5/7. How many millilitres of cough mixture should the pharmacist dispense?

Volume used per day is:

2.0 mL × 3 = 6.0 mL

5/7 means 5 days, therefore the total volume used is:

5 × 6 mL = 30 mL

The pharmacist should dispense 30 mL.

Doses based on the weight of drug

Solid formulations

In most official publications the dose of a drug is a specified weight or weight range, which may be accompanied by other instructions such as time intervals between doses, specified times of administration, length of treatment, etc. For example, the dose of domperidone by mouth is 10–20 mg every 4–8 hours, with a maximum period of treatment of 12 weeks.

Many drugs are available in one or more formulations and may be available in one or more strengths. For example, domperidone is available as a 10 mg tablet, as a suppository containing 30 mg and as a suspension containing 5 mg in 5 mL. A pharmacist may therefore be required to convert a dose of a drug into an equivalent number of tablets, suppositories or another dosage form.

EXAMPLE 6.6

A prescription requires a patient to receive 20 mg domperidone (in tablet form) every 8 hours for 4 weeks. How many tablets should the pharmacist dispense?

Domperidone tablets are only available as 10 mg tablets, therefore in order for the patient to receive a dose of 20 mg, he or she will need to take two 10 mg tablets. Every 8 hours is equivalent to three times a day, therefore the patient will need to take 6 tablets per day.

Four weeks is:

$$4 \times 7 \text{ days} = 28 \text{ days}$$

Total number of 10 mg tablets is:

$$6 \times 28 = 168$$

The pharmacist should dispense 168 tablets.

On occasions, two strengths of the same medicinal product have to be used to obtain the correct dose. Example 6.7 demonstrates such a situation.

EXAMPLE 6.7

A patient requires 8 mg of prednisolone per day for 1 week followed by 7 mg of prednisolone per day for the next week. Prednisolone is available in tablets of 1 mg and 5 mg. How many tablets of each strength should the pharmacist supply?

8 mg of prednisolone could be supplied by one 5 mg tablet and three 1 mg tablets, therefore 1 week's supply would consist of seven 5 mg tablets and twenty-one 1 mg tablets.

7 mg of prednisolone could be supplied by one 5 mg tablet and two 1 mg tablets, therefore 1 week's supply would consist of seven 5 mg tablets and fourteen 1 mg tablets.

Thus, the total quantities supplied by the pharmacist should be fourteen 5 mg tablets and thirty-five 1 mg tablets.

In Examples 6.6 and 6.7 only tablets have been used to illustrate the basic calculations. However, in practice similar calculations could involve suppositories, capsules, powders or other solid dosage forms.

Liquid formulations

In a similar way to solid formulations, liquid formulations may be prescribed using the weight of the drug as the dose. For example, a prescription may state 120 mg of paracetamol to be taken twice a day supplied as a suspension. Paracetamol oral suspension contains 120 mg of paracetamol in each 5 mL. Thus, each dose would be 5 mL and the patient would be instructed to take one 5 mL spoonful twice a day.

If the dose is expressed as the weight of drug, then in the case of a liquid formulation, the dose taken by the patient may be 5 mL or a multiple thereof. Example 6.8 illustrates such a situation.

EXAMPLE 6.8

A prescription requires 300 mg of paracetamol to be taken four times a day for 3 days, supplied as paracetamol 120 mg/5 mL suspension. Calculate the volume of paracetamol suspension to be supplied.

First it is necessary to find out what volume of suspension contains 300 mg of paracetamol. We know the suspension contains 120 mg/5 mL.

Let the unknown volume of suspension that contains 300 mg be *y*. Setting up proportional sets:

weight of paracetamol (mg)	300	120
volume of suspension (mL)	*y*	5

$$\frac{y}{300} = \frac{5}{120}$$

$$y = \frac{5 \times 300}{120}$$

$$y = 12.5$$

The volume of suspension that contains 300 mg is 12.5 mL, therefore a dose of 12.5 mL four times a day for 3 days would need to be supplied. The total volume to be supplied is:

$$12.5 \times 4 \times 3 = 150 \text{ mL}$$

If a liquid formulation is prescribed for a very frail person or a very young child, then the dose required may be less than 5 mL. Example 6.9 demonstrates such a situation.

EXAMPLE 6.9

A prescription requires a dose of 30 mg of paracetamol. What volume of paracetamol suspension would provide a dose of 30 mg?

We know that paracetamol suspension contains 120 mg/5 mL.
Let the unknown volume of suspension be *y*. Setting up proportional sets:

weight of paracetamol (mg)	120	30
volume of suspension (mL)	5	*y*

$$\frac{y}{30} = \frac{5}{120}$$

$$y = \frac{5 \times 30}{120}$$

$$y = 1.25$$

1.25 mL of paracetamol suspension contains 30 mg of paracetamol.

Injections are another form of liquid formulation. In some situations the dose required may be expressed as a weight and thus the dose will have to be converted to a suitable volume, as in Example 6.10.

EXAMPLE 6.10

A patient requires an emergency loading dose of 0.5 mg of digoxin. Digoxin is available as an injection containing 250 micrograms/mL. How many millilitres of injection will supply the required dose? [Note: do not confuse micrograms with milligrams.]

First convert 0.5 mg to micrograms using the place value approach:

$$mg \quad - \quad - \quad micrograms$$

$$0.5 \text{ mg} = \quad 0 \quad 5 \quad 0 \quad 0 \qquad = 500 \text{ micrograms}$$

Let the required volume of digoxin injection be y. Setting up proportional sets:

weight of digoxin (micrograms)	250	500
volume of injection (mL)	1	y

We can spot that 250 is multiplied by 2 to give 500, so 1 is multiplied by 2 to give y.
The patient should receive 2 mL of digoxin injection, which will contain 0.5 mg (500 micrograms) of digoxin.

Doses based on body weight

Many drugs are potent and the dose of such drugs will take into account the body weight of the person receiving the drug. It is therefore common

Table 6.1 Age and related body weight and height

Age	Ideal body weight (kg)	Height (cm)
Newborn*	3.4	50
1 month*	4.2	55
3 months*	5.6	59
6 months	7.7	67
1 year	10	76
3 years	14	94
5 years	18	108
7 years	23	120
12 years	37	148
Adult male	68	173
Adult female	56	163

*These figures relate to full-term but not preterm infants, who may need reduced dosage according to their clinical condition.

to express the dose as the weight of drug per kilogram of body weight. In particular this method is used for children, since the body weight of children will depend on a number of factors, including age and state of health. Average body weights are given in Table 6.1.

From Table 6.1 it can be seen that the average adult male is considered to have a body weight of 68 kg and the average adult female to have a body weight of 56 kg, although there will be considerable variation about these average weights. The body weights of children can also be obtained from Table 6.1. For example, a 6-month-old child weighs on average 7.7 kg and a 5-year-old child weighs on average 18 kg. If the child's age is not given in the table, it is usual to estimate the body weight using the weights on either side of the age of the child or to take into account the height of the child. For example, the body weight of a 4-year-old child would be estimated to be between that of a 3-year old and a 5-year-old, that is about 16 kg. In the case of an exceptionally tall or short child it may be more appropriate to estimate the dose using height.

The calculation of a dose based on body weight may produce a value that does not correspond to an available dosage form. Example 6.11 illustrates such a situation.

EXAMPLE 6.11

Calculate the dose of ketoconazole for a child of 3 years of age and a child of 11 years. Suggest a suitable formulation for both. The recommended dose of ketoconazole is 3 mg/kg daily.

3-year-old child

From Table 6.1, a 3-year-old child weighs 14 kg.

Let the daily dose in milligrams be y. Setting up proportional sets:

dose of ketoconazole (mg) 3 y

body weight (kg)   1   14

$$y = 3 \times 14$$

$$y = 42$$

The daily dose for a 3-year-old child is 42 mg.

This dose has to be translated into a suitable formulation for a child. The available formulations of ketoconazole are scored tablets of 200 mg and a suspension containing ketoconazole 100 mg/5 mL. Clearly, if the recommended dose is 42 mg, then the 200 mg tablets are not suitable. (Also remember that a 3-year-old child may not be able to swallow tablets.) The suspension is a suitable product, but a 5 mL dose contains 100 mg of ketoconazole. It is therefore necessary to calculate the volume of suspension that contains the correct dose.

Let the required volume of ketoconazole suspension (mL) be y. Setting up proportional sets:

dose of ketoconazole (mg)   42   100

volume of suspension (mL) y 5

$$\frac{y}{42} = \frac{5}{100}$$

$$y = \frac{5 \times 42}{100}$$

$$y = 2.1$$

The child should be given 2.1 mL of ketoconazole suspension per day.

11-year-old child

Table 6.1 only gives weights for a 7-year-old and a 12-year-old, therefore the body weight has to be estimated. In this case the estimate is about 34 kg.

Let the daily dose of ketoconazole (mg) be z. Setting up proportional sets:

daily dose of ketoconazole (mg)   3 z

body weight (kg)   1   34

$z = 102$

The daily dose for an 11-year-old child is 102 mg.

Again it is necessary to translate this dose into a suitable formulation. Since the body weight of the child was estimated, it is possible to reduce (or round off) the dose to a convenient 100 mg. In this situation an 11-year-old child might be capable of swallowing a tablet, depending on their medical condition. For a dose of 102 mg it would be possible to halve the 200 mg tablet (it is a scored tablet) and give the child half a tablet (the equivalent of approximately 100 mg). Alternatively, a 5 mL dose of the suspension containing 100 mg/5 mL could be given.

Example 6.11 used a drug with a daily dose. Some drugs need to be given at more frequent intervals, as in Example 6.12.

EXAMPLE 6.12

The drug nitrofurantoin has dose of 3 mg/kg daily in four divided doses for children over 3 months. Calculate the dose for a 5-year-old child and recommend a suitable dosage form.

From Table 6.1, a 5-year-old child weighs 18 kg.

Let the daily dose in milligrams be y. Setting up proportional sets:

daily dose of nitrofurantoin (mg)   3 y

body weight (kg)   1   18

$y = 3 \times 18$

$y = 54$

The daily dose is 54 mg. This daily dose has to be converted into four doses per day, that is 54 mg divided by 4, which is 13.5 mg. The dosage regimen is therefore 13.5 mg four times per day.

The available formulations of nitrofurantoin are 50 mg and 100 mg tablets, and a suspension containing 25 mg/5 mL. Clearly the tablets are not suitable and therefore the suspension must be used. A 5 mL dose of the suspension contains 25 mg but the required dose is 13.5 mg.

Let the required volume of suspension be y. Setting up proportional sets:

volume of suspension (mL)	5	y
dose of nitrofurantoin (mg)	25	13.5

We can spot that 25 is divided by 5 to give 5, therefore 13.5 is divided by 5 to give 2.7.

Alternatively:

$$y = \frac{5 \times 13.5}{25}$$

$$y = 2.7$$

The child should be given 2.7 mL of nitrofurantoin suspension four times a day.

Many drugs can be given by injection and some of the doses of these injectable drugs may be calculated using body weight, as in Example 6.13.

EXAMPLE 6.13

The drug gentamicin has a dose of 2 mg/kg every 8 hours for children between 2 weeks and 12 years of age. Calculate the dose for a 6-month-old child and the volume of paediatric injection to be given.

From Table 6.1, a 6-month-old child weighs 7.7 kg.

Let the required dose be y. Setting up proportional sets:

dose of gentamicin (mg)	2	y
body weight (kg)	1	7.7

We can spot that 1 is multiplied by 2 to give 2, so 7.7 is multiplied by 2 to give 15.4.

Alternatively:

$$y = \frac{2 \times 7.7}{1}$$

$$y = 15.4$$

The dose of gentamicin is 15.4 mg.

The paediatric injection contains gentamicin 10 mg/mL.

Let the required volume of injection be z. Setting up proportional sets:

volume of injection (mL)	1	z
amount of gentamicin (mg)	10	15.4

$$z = \frac{15.4}{10}$$

$$z = 1.54$$

1.54 mL of injection should be administered every 8 hours.

. . . .

Doses based on body surface area

The doses of some drugs (not many) are expressed as the quantity of drug per metre squared of body surface area. Examples of such drugs are methotrexate, zidovudine (children only) and lomustine. Paediatric doses may be estimated more accurately using the body surface area method, since many physiological phenomena correlate better to body surface area. The calculation of doses using body surface area of necessity must involved determining or obtaining the body surface area. Table 6.2 shows the body surface areas for different ages. More accurate estimates of body surface area can be obtained using published nomograms.

The method of calculation of doses using body surface area is similar to that using body weight. In other words, the body surface area must be found from the table before the dose can be calculated, then a suitable dosage form must be found that will deliver the dose.

Table 6.2 Age and body surface area

Age	Body surface area (m²)
Newborn*	0.23
1 month*	0.26
3 months*	0.32
6 months	0.40
1 year	0.47
3 years	0.62
5 years	0.73
7 years	0.88
12 years	1.25
Adult male	1.80
Adult female	1.60

*These figures relate to full-term but not preterm infants who may need reduced dosage according to their clinical condition.

EXAMPLE 6.14

Calculate the oral dose of methotrexate suitable for a 12-year-old child and suggest a suitable dosage form. The oral dose of methotrexate is 15 mg/m² weekly. Methotrexate tablets are available as 2.5 mg and 10 mg.

The body surface area of a 12-year-old child is 1.25 m².
   Let the weekly dose of methotrexate be y. Setting up proportional sets:

dose of methotrexate (mg)   15 y

body surface area (m²)   1   1.25

Spotting the relationship between 15 and 1, 1.25 is multiplied by 15 to give y:

$$y = 18.75$$

The weekly dose of methotrexate is 18.75 mg.
In order to provide 18.25 mg from these two available tablets, the patient would need to take one 10 mg tablet and three and a half 2.5 mg tablets.

Since the body surface method is more accurate than other methods of dose calculation, it is possible to estimate a dose for a child from a published adult dose, if a paediatric dose is not available. However, remember that if a paediatric dose is not available, then that drug is probably not licensed for use in children.

EXAMPLE 6.15

Calculate the dose of drug X for a 7-year-old male child, using the body surface method, assuming that the adult dose is 50 mg daily.

The body surface area for an adult and for a 7-year-old child are 1.8 and 0.88 m², respectively.

Let the required paediatric dose be y. Setting up proportional sets:

dose (mg) y 50

surface area (m²)   0.88   1.8

$$y = \frac{50 \times 0.88}{1.8}$$

$y = 24.4$

The required child dose is 24.4 mg daily.

Doses as a percentage of the adult dose

Doses for children of commonly prescribed drugs that have a wide margin of error between the therapeutic dose and the toxic dose can be calculated using the percentage of the adult dose method. Again a table showing the relationship between age and percentage of the adult dose is available (Table 6.3).

EXAMPLE 6.16

Calculate the dose of drug X for a 5-year-old child. The adult daily dose of drug X is 325 mg.

From Table 6.3, a 5-year-old child should be given 40% of the adult dose.

Let the required dose for a 5-year-old child be y.

Table 6.3 Relationship between age and percentage of adult dose

Age	Percentage of adult dose
Newborn*	12.5
1 month*	14.5
3 months*	18
6 months	22
1 year	25
3 years	33
5 years	40
7 years	50
12 years	75

*The figures relate to full-term and not preterm infants who may need reduced dosage according to their clinical condition.

Setting up proportional sets:

$$\text{dose (mg)} \quad y \quad 325$$

$$\text{percentage} \quad 40 \quad 100$$

$$\frac{y}{40} = \frac{325}{100}$$

$$y = \frac{325 \times 40}{100}$$

$$y = 130$$

The dose for a 5-year-old child using the percentage method is 130 mg per day.

Doses based on units

The doses of some drugs, usually large biological molecules, are expressed in units rather than weights. Such large molecules are difficult to purify and so rather than use a weight it is more accurate to use the biological activity of the drug. The biological activity is expressed in units. Examples of such drugs are some hormone products, insulin and a few anti-infective drugs.

The calculation of doses and translation into suitable dosage forms are similar to the calculations elsewhere in this chapter.

EXAMPLE 6.17

The antifungal drug nystatin has a recommended oral dose for adults of 500 000 units every 6 hours, doubled in severe infection for the treatment of candidiasis. Tablets containing 500 000 units and a suspension containing 100 000 units/mL are available. Assuming an adult had a severe infection, what dose of nystatin should be recommended and what quantities of both available formulations would be required for 5 days of treatment?

The adult dose in the case of a severe infection is twice the normal dose, that is 1 000 000 units every 6 hours (in other words four times a day). Each tablet contains 500 000 units, so the dose is two tablets. The patient requires four doses of two tablets per day = 8 tablets, therefore the total number of tablets for 5 days is:

$$5 \times 8 = 40$$

The patient will therefore require 40 tablets of nystatin for the course of treatment.

The patient could also be prescribed the suspension, which contains 100 000 units per millilitre. Each dose contains 1 000 000 units, therefore each dose of suspension would be:

$$\frac{1\,000\,000}{100\,000} = 10\,\text{mL}$$

Again the patient requires four doses of 10 mL per day = 40 mL, therefore the total volume of suspension for 5 days = 5 × 40 = 200 mL.

Practice calculations

Answers are given at the end of the chapter.

Q1 A patient is prescribed two tablets of drug A four times a day for 3 months. How many tablets of drug A should the pharmacist dispense?

Q2 A customer buys an over-the-counter pack of 100 vitamin capsules. The dosage regimen is one capsule three times a day. How many days will the pack last if the customer takes the capsules according to the dosage regimen?

Q3   An inhaler contains 200 metered doses. If the patient inhales two doses three times a day, how long will the inhaler last?

Q4   A patient is prescribed analgesic suppositories to be used six times a day for 5 days, then three times a day for 3 days. How many suppositories should the pharmacist dispense?

Q5   A patient going to a high-risk malaria area requires 8 weeks treatment. Two different antimalarial tablets are prescribed, A and B. Drug A has a dosage regimen of one tablet per week and drug B has a dosage regimen of two tablets daily. How many tablets of A and B should be supplied to cover the period the patient is in the malaria area?

Q6   A residential home buys a 1000 pack of senna tablets. Each resident is given two tablets each night. There are 35 residents. How long will it take to use all the senna tablets?

Q7   A prescription for charcoal sachets reads:

Two sachets three times a day for 1/12

How many sachets should be supplied?

Q8   A prescription for drug Y reads:

Three capsules twice a day for 3/7

Two capsules twice a day for 3/7

One capsule twice a day for 2/52

How many capsules should the pharmacist dispense?

Q9   A sachet of normal saline solution is used to bathe an eye. A patient is instructed to bathe both eyes twice a day for 1/12. How many sachets should be supplied to the patient?

Q10   A patient is going on holiday for 3 weeks. He is supplied with 168 tablets of drug C. The dosage regimen is two tablets four times a day. Will the patient have sufficient tablets for the duration of his holiday?

Q11   A patient uses nicotine patches at the rate of one patch every 3 days. How many patches will the patient require for 3 months?

Q12   A patient pack of a drug contains 56 tablets. If the dosage regimen is one tablet four times a day for 4 weeks, how many packs should the pharmacist supply?

Q13   A patient pack of a drug contains 84 tablets and is designed to last for 1 month. If the patient takes one dose twice a day, what is the dose?

Q14   How many 5 mL doses are contained in 120 mL of mixture?

Q15   A patient is required to use 30 mL of mouthwash twice a day. What volume of mouthwash should the pharmacist supply for a 14-day course of treatment?

Q16   A prescription for an indigestion mixture reads:

>   15 mL four times a day for 2/52

How much mixture should the pharmacist dispense?

Q17   How many 15 mL doses are contained in 240 mL of mixture?

Q18   A patient takes 10 mL of laxative solution at night. What volume will the patient use in a month?

Q19   A mother buys a 150 mL bottle of cough elixir. She gives each of her two children 5 mL four times a day for 3 days. How many doses will be left at the end of 3 days?

Q20   A prescription for a young child reads:

>   2.5 mL three times a day for 4/7

What volume of drug should the pharmacist dispense?

Q21   A patient requires 7.5 mL of a mixture to be taken four times a day for 3/52. What volume of mixture should be supplied?

Q22   A patient pack contains 30 mL of a syrup. How many days will the syrup last for if the dose is 0.5 mL three times a day?

Q23 A scored tablet containing 100 mg of drug X is available. A prescription for drug X reads:

> 50 mg three times a day for 10 days

How many tablets should the pharmacist dispense?

Q24 Drug Z is only available as a capsule containing 62.5 mg. A prescription reads:

> 125 mg four times a day for 1/12

How many capsules of drug Z should the pharmacist dispense?

Q25 Drug A is available as a tablet containing 500 micrograms. A patient requires 2 mg of drug A four times a day for 3/7 and 1.5 mg of drug A for 5/7. How many tablets of drug will be required for a dose of 2 mg and a dose of 1.5 mg? Calculate the total number of tablets to be dispensed to fill the prescription.

Q26 A prescription for drug B reads:

> 500 mg twice a day for 5 days

Drug B is available as a capsules containing 250 mg. How many capsules should be dispensed to fill the prescription?

Q27 Drug A is available as 2.5 mg and 5 mg tablets. A prescription for drug A requires:

> 7.5 mg three times a day for 5 days, then
>
> 5 mg four times a day for 3 days, then
>
> 5 mg twice a day for 3 days, then
>
> 2.5 mg three times a day for 7 days

Calculate how many tablets of 5 mg and 2.5 mg are required to fill the prescription.

Q28 A prescription for drug Z reads:

> 62.5 mg three times a day for 5 days

Drug Z is available as a suspension containing 250 mg/5 mL. Calculate the volume of each dose and calculate the volume of suspension that should be supplied to the patient.

Q29 A prescription for drug X reads:

> 240 mg four times a day. Send 100 mL of mixture

Drug X is available as a mixture containing 120 mg/5 mL. Calculate for how many days the mixture will last, assuming the mixture is taken according to the dosage regimen.

Q30 A solution contains 500 units per millilitre and the pack size is 25 mL. A patient is given 2500 units three times a day for 5 days. How many packs should the pharmacist dispense for the patient?

Q31 Drug A is available as an elixir containing 150 mg/5 mL. A prescription reads:

> 225 mg four times a day for 7 days

What volume of the elixir should the pharmacist supply?

Q32 A patient requires 15 mg of morphine sulphate by subcutaneous injection every 4 hours for 16 hours. Morphine sulphate injection is available as 20 mg/1 mL. What volume of injection should be given on each dosing occasion? What is the total quantity of morphine sulphate given over the 16 hours?

Q33 The dose of morphine sulphate for a 6-month-old child by subcutaneous injection is 200 micrograms/kg. Calculate the quantity of morphine sulphate required for one dose. What volume of injection should be administered, assuming it is available in a concentration of 10 mg/mL?

Q34 Pethidine hydrochloride injection is available in 100 mg/2 mL ampoules. The recommended dose for a child by intramuscular injection is 0.5–2 mg/kg. Calculate both extremes of this dose range for a 12-year-old child. What volume of injection solution should be administered for both these doses?

Q35 The recommended oral dose for a child of griseofulvin is 10 mg/kg daily. A suspension containing griseofulvin 125 mg/5 mL is available. Calculate the dose for a 5-year-old child and the volume of suspension to be given per dose.

Q36 Using the information in question 35, calculate the oral dose of griseofulvin and the volume of suspension required for a 12-year-old child.

Q37 The recommended dose of didanosine is $120\ mg/m^2$ every 12 hours. Calculate the dose and daily dose for a 7-year-old child.

Q38 Drug X has a recommended oral dose for a 6-month-old child of 8 mg/kg twice a day. A suspension is available at a concentration of 40 mg/5 mL. Calculate the dose for a 6-month-old child and recommend the volume of suspension to be administered at each dose.

Q39 The adult dose of drug X is 75 mg daily. Using the body surface method, calculate the dose for a 5-year-old child.

Q40 Using the data given in question 39, calculate the dose of drug X for a 10-year-old child.

Q41 The recommended oral dose of hydroxychloroquine sulphate for a child is 6.5 mg/kg daily. Calculate the dose for a 7-year-old child.

Q42 The adult oral dose of hydroxychloroquine sulphate is 200–400 mg daily. Use the percentage of adult dose method to estimate the dose for a 7-year-old child. Compare your results by this method with your answer for question 41.

Q43 The adult dose of drug C is 50 micrograms. Calculate the dose for a 3-year-old child by the body surface method and the percentage of adult dose method. Compare your two answers.

Answers

A1 672

A2 33.3 rounded to 33 days

A3 33.3 rounded to 33 days

A4 39

A5 8 tablets of drug A
112 tablets of drug B

A6 14.28 rounded to 14 days

A7   168

A8   58

A9   112

A10   Yes

A11   28

A12   2

A13   1.5 tablets

A14   24

A15   840 mL

A16   840 mL

A17   16

A18   280 mL

A19   6

A20   30 mL

A21   630 mL

A22   20 days

A23   15

A24   224

A25   4, 3, 63

A26   20

A27   Thirty-three 5 mg tablets
         Thirty-six 2.5 mg tablets

A28 1.25 mL dose
18.75 mL total volume

A29 2.5 days

A30 Three

A31 210 mL

A32 0.75 mL per dose
75 mg (every 4 hours for 16 hours is five doses)

A33 1.54 mg
0.154 mL

A34 18.5–74 mg
0.37–1.48 mL

A35 180 mg
7.2 mL

A36 370 mg
14.8 mL

A37 105.6 mg
211.2 mg

A38 61.6 mg twice a day
7.7 mL

A39 30.4 mg

A40 41.7 mg

A41 149.5 mg

A42 100–200 mg daily

A43 17.2 micrograms
16.5 micrograms

7

Displacement volumes and values, and density

Displacement volumes involving solids in liquids

If we add 5 mL of water to 95 mL of water then we will have a total volume of 100 mL of water. However, if we add 5 g of salt to 95 mL of water and stir the mixture until the salt has dissolved, then we will have a total volume of solution above 95 mL, but it is unlikely to be exactly 100 mL: it may be less than 100 mL or it may be greater. The 5 g of salt dissolves in the water and increases the total volume. In other words, the salt occupies a space and displaces some of the water such that the total volume of the solution is more than 95 mL. This phenomenon in which the salt displaces some of the water and results in an increase in the volume of the resulting solution is important in pharmacy and has resulted in the determination and publication of displacement volumes.

A displacement volume is the quantity of solvent that is displaced by a specified quantity of a solid during dissolution. It is the space or volume of solvent that is occupied by the solute after a solution has been produced. For example, chloramphenicol powder for reconstitution into an injection has a displacement volume of 0.8 mL/g. This means that 1 g of chloramphenicol powder will displace (or occupy the space of) 0.8 mL when it is dissolved in water.

The correct use of displacement volumes is essential when water for injection or other suitable diluent is added to drug powder in order to produce an injection solution of a known concentration and volume. For example, the displacement volume of diamorphine is quoted as 0.06 mL/5 mg. This means that 5 mg of diamorphine will displace (or occupy the volume of) 0.06 mL of water. This information can be used to calculate the correct volume of water for injection to add to diamorphine powder to make a known volume of injection solution at a known concentration. This is illustrated in Example 7.1.

EXAMPLE 7.1

Calculate the volume of water for injection required to produce 1 mL of an injection containing 5 mg diamorphine. A vial containing 5 mg of diamorphine powder (suitable for reconstitution into an injection) and water for injection is available. The displacement volume of diamorphine is 0.06 mL/5 mg.

The final volume is specified as 1 mL and the volume occupied by the powder is obtained from the displacement volume. The displacement volume is 0.06 mL/5 mg and so the volume occupied by 5 mg of powder will be equivalent to 0.06 mL. The volume of water required is therefore:

$$1 - 0.06 = 0.94 \text{ mL}$$

Now calculate what would happen if the pharmacist ignored the displacement volume and added 1 mL of water to the powder instead of 0.94 mL. 5 mg of the diamorphine powder displaces 0.06 mL of water, therefore if 1 mL of water is added to the powder the total volume of the solution will be:

$$1 + 0.06 = 1.06 \text{ mL}$$

The difference between 1 mL and 1.06 mL may appear small but it will dilute the concentration of the drug, and if the patient was administered 1 mL (as the prescriber requested) then the patient would not receive the correct dose. The dose administered would be 4.7 mg as opposed to the 5 mg requested.

Let us try another example, involving the determination of the volume required to produce the correct concentration of the drug.

EXAMPLE 7.2

The displacement volume of drug X is 0.5 mL/50 mg. Drug X is required at a concentration of 4 mg in 1 mL. Calculate the volume of diluent that must be added to 50 mg of drug X to produce the required concentration.

First determine the final volume of the drug solution. Let the final volume be y. Setting up proportional sets:

amount of drug (mg)	4	50
volume (mL)	1	y

We can spot that 4 divided by 4 gives 1, so 50 divided by 4 gives y, therefore:

$$y = 12.5$$

The final volume of the solution will be 12.5 mL, and this volume will contain 50 mg of drug X.

We know that the volume of diluent required for the reconstitution of drug X is the final volume minus the displacement volume of 50 mg of the drug. Since the displacement volume of drug X is 0.5 mL/50 mg, then the required volume of diluent is:

$$12.5 - 0.5 = 12.0 \text{ mL}$$

A table of displacement volumes of powder injections is published in *The Pharmaceutical Codex*. This table, however, only gives the displacement volume for one specific quantity of each drug. For example, in the case of diamorphine the displacement volume is that quoted above (0.06 mL/5 mg). Diamorphine is available as a powder for reconstitution in quantities greater than 5 mg. If the prescriber requires more than 5 mg, then these other quantities of powders will need to be used. In such cases it will be necessary to calculate a displacement volume for another quantity of diamorphine.

EXAMPLE 7.3

Diamorphine is available as a powder for reconstitution in quantities of 30 mg, 100 mg and 500 mg. Using the displacement volume of 0.06 mL/5 mg, calculate how much diluent will be displaced by 30 mg, 100 mg and 500 mg of diamorphine.

Let the volumes displaced by 30 mg, 100 mg and 500 mg, respectively, be x, y and z. Setting up proportional sets:

volume (mL)	0.06	x	y	z
diamorphine (mg)	5	30	100	500

We can find the values of x, y and z by spotting the relationship between 5 and 30, and 100 and 500.

Alternatively:

$$\frac{0.06}{5} = \frac{x}{30} = \frac{y}{100} = \frac{z}{500}$$

therefore:

$x = 0.36$

$y = 1.2$

$z = 6.0$

30 mg, 100 mg and 500 mg of diamorphine will displace, respectively, 0.36 mL, 1.2 mL and 6.0 mL of diluent.

....

Let us now consider displacement volumes in a different way. Many antibiotics are liable to hydrolysis when mixed with water. However, small children cannot take antibiotic tablets or capsules and so, rather than prescribe an antibiotic injection, prescribers may request an antibiotic mixture. Such an antibiotic mixture will have a short time span before the antibiotic is hydrolysed. The pharmacist will therefore prepare the mixture at the time the prescription is presented. Most commercial antibiotic mixture preparations consist of an antibiotic powder mix to which the pharmacist has to add a specific volume of water to produce an exact volume of mixture at a known concentration. This specified volume of water will depend on the manufacturer assuming a displacement volume for the antibiotic powder mix.

EXAMPLE 7.4

In order to produce 100 mL of a mixture containing 125 mg of antibiotic A in each 5 mL dose, the pharmacist is required to add 68 mL of water to the antibiotic powder mix. Calculate the displacement volume for a quantity of powder equivalent to 125 mg of antibiotic A.

We need to calculate the total amount of antibiotic in the 100 mL of final mixture. After reconstitution there will be 125 mg of antibiotic A in 5 mL.

Let the total amount of antibiotic A in 100 mL be y. Setting up proportional sets:

amount of antibiotic A (mg)	125	y
volume (mL)	5	100

We can spot that 5 is multiplied by 25 to give 125, so 100 is multiplied by 25 to give y, therefore:

$$y = 2500$$

100 mL of the final mixture contains 2500 mg of antibiotic A.

If the pharmacist has to add 68 mL of water to the antibiotic powder mix to produce a final volume of 100 mL, then the antibiotic powder mix must displace 32 mL of water, i.e. 100 − 68 mL. Thus, the antibiotic powder mix contains 2500 mg of antibiotic A and this displaces 32 mL of water.

To calculate the displacement volume of this powder mix, let the volume displaced by antibiotic powder mix, equivalent to 125 mg of antibiotic A, be x. Setting up proportional sets:

volume (mL)	32	x
antibiotic (mg)	2500	125

$$\frac{32}{2500} = \frac{x}{125}$$

$$x = \frac{32 \times 125}{2500}$$

$$x = 1.6$$

1.6 mL of water is therefore displaced by a quantity of antibiotic powder mix containing 125 mg of antibiotic A.

Displacement values involving solids incorporated into other solids

In order to understand displacement values involving solids incorporated into other solids, we need to consider what is meant by the term 'bulk density'. Compare two objects, a metal coin and a bath sponge. If we consider the weight of each, then the sponge is probably lighter than the coin, but look at the difference in volume. The coin is very small and the bath sponge is probably at least 100 times larger. The coin, which is metallic, is very dense and has a high bulk density, i.e. 1 g of the metal occupies a small space. In contrast, the sponge is comparatively light in weight for its size compared to the coin and occupies a larger space. The sponge therefore has a low bulk density. This concept of the different bulk densities of different drugs is used in calculations involving the preparation of suppositories and pessaries.

Calculations for suppositories and pessaries

Extemporaneously prepared suppositories and pessaries involve incorporating a drug or drugs into either a waxy or, less frequently, a glyco gelatin base. The process involves the use of a mould so that the size of the suppository is the same irrespective of which base or drug(s) is used in the preparation. The mould contains a known volume and weight of the base. In the preparation of suppositories the base is mixed with the drug. However, the base and drug may have different bulk densities, therefore a drug with a low bulk density will displace more of the base than a similar weight of a drug with a high bulk density. In order to ensure that each suppository contains the correct amount of the drug, the bulk density of the drug has to be taken into account. For many drugs that would be incorporated into a suppository base, the weights that would displace 1 g of the traditional suppository base (theobroma oil) have been calculated and published in *The Pharmaceutical Codex*. These values are referred to as *displacement values*.

For example, the displacement value of zinc oxide is 4.7. This means that 4.7 g of zinc oxide will displace (or occupy the space of) 1 g of theobroma oil (the suppository or pessary base). In other words, zinc oxide is much denser than theobroma oil. Another example is menthol, which has a displacement value of 0.7. This means that 0.7 g of menthol will displace 1 g of theobroma oil. In this case menthol is less dense than the suppository base.

In order to calculate the amount of base to be added to the drug to provide the correct amount of drug in each suppository, the displacement value must be used. However, it should be noted that a displacement value is only used when the drug is expressed as an actual quantity, for example x mg or y g.

(Suppository and pessary moulds are produced in nominal sizes of 1 g, 2 g, etc. The nominal mould size refers to the quantity of theobroma oil that would occupy the mould. Before use a pharmacist should calibrate the mould by filling with theobroma oil and weighing the suppository produced. The weight of the suppository will indicate the actual size of the mould. If this is substantially different to the nominal value, then the actual value should be used in the calculations shown below.)

Waxy or oily bases

In the previous section theobroma oil was said to be the traditional suppository base. Theobroma oil is a natural waxy material that is solid at room temperature and melts at body temperature, i.e. when inserted into a body cavity. However, in recent years synthetic suppository bases have been developed that have almost replaced the use of theobroma oil. Most of the modern synthetic bases have similar density properties to theobroma oil and so the displacement values determined for drugs incorporated into theobroma oil can be used for the modern synthetic bases.

Displacement values have to be used to calculate the amount of suppository base required when a specified amount of a drug has to be incorporated into a suppository.

EXAMPLE 7.5

A pharmacist has to prepare six suppositories for a patient, each suppository to be made in a nominal 1 g mould and to contain 0.3 g of zinc oxide. Calculate the amount of the base (theobroma oil) that the pharmacist will need to use. Assume that due to the method of preparation the pharmacist will need to make an excess of the mixture and so it will be necessary to calculate the quantities for the preparation of eight suppositories.

The displacement value of zinc oxide is 4.7 and hence 4.7 g of zinc oxide will displace 1 g of base. We need to calculate how much zinc oxide is required for the eight suppositories and how much base will be displaced by that quantity of zinc oxide. Each suppository contains 0.3 g zinc oxide.

For eight suppositories the total amount of zinc oxide will be $8 \times 0.3 = 2.4$ g.

Let the amount of base displaced by 2.4 g of zinc oxide be y. Setting up proportional sets:

mass of zinc oxide (g)	4.7	2.4
base displaced (g)	1	y

$$\frac{y}{2.4} = \frac{1}{4.7}$$

$$y = 0.51$$

2.4 g of zinc oxide will displace 0.51 g of suppository base.

If the pharmacist is preparing eight suppositories of 1 g each then the amount of base required will be the amount of base needed to fill eight moulds minus the weight of base displaced by the zinc oxide:

$$(8 \times 1) - 0.51 = 7.49 \text{ g of base}$$

Thus, the final composition of the suppository mixture will be:

zinc oxide	2.4 g
suppository base	7.49 g
total weight	9.89 g

Note that the total weight is greater than the nominal weight of eight suppositories, i.e. 8×1 g. This weight difference is because the displacement value of zinc oxide is greater than 1.

Example 7.6 demonstrates the situation when the displacement value is less than 1.

EXAMPLE 7.6

Calculate the quantities required to prepare sufficient suppository mixture for twelve 1 g suppositories each containing 50 mg of menthol in theobroma oil. What will each suppository weigh? Assume no excess mixture is needed.

The displacement value of menthol is 0.7. The displacement value is expressed in terms of grams, so the 50 mg dose of menthol has to be converted into grams:

$$g \quad - \quad - \quad mg$$
$$50\ mg = \quad 0 \quad 0 \quad 5 \quad 0 \quad = 0.05\ g$$

12 suppositories will contain 0.6 g of menthol.

Let the amount of base displaced by the menthol in 12 suppositories be y. Setting up proportional sets:

mass of menthol (g)	0.7	0.6
base displaced (g)	1	y

$y = 0.86$

0.6 g of menthol displaces 0.86 g of theobroma base, therefore the quantity of theobroma oil required to produce 12 suppositories, containing a total of 0.6 g of menthol, is:

$(12 \times 1) - 0.86 = 11.14\ g$

The final formula for 12 suppositories is:

menthol	0.6 g
theobroma oil	11.14 g
total weight	11.74 g

therefore each suppository weighs 0.98 g. This is less than the nominal 1 g because of the displacement value for the menthol.

If more than one medicament is included in a suppository, then the displacement of the base caused by both medicaments should be calculated.

EXAMPLE 7.7

Assume the menthol suppositories in Example 7.6 have each to contain 300 mg of paracetamol in addition to the menthol. Calculate the weight of base required to produce the same quantity of suppository mixture.

First calculate the amount of base displaced by the paracetamol. Each suppository will contain 300 mg (0.3 g) of paracetamol and 12 suppositories will contain 12 × 0.3 g = 3.6 g of paracetamol. The displacement value of paracetamol is 1.5.

Let the amount of base displaced by 3.6 g of paracetamol be b. Setting up proportional sets:

mass of paracetamol (g)	1.5	3.6
base displaced (g)	1	b

$$\frac{b}{3.6} = \frac{1}{1.5}$$

$$b = 2.4$$

3.6 g of paracetamol displaces 2.4 g of suppository base.

The amount of base required to produce the suppositories is 12 × 1 g minus the amounts displaced by both the menthol and the paracetamol. Remember that the menthol will displace 0.86 g of base and the paracetamol will displace 2.4 g.

The weight of base required is:

$$12 - (0.86 + 2.4) = 8.74 \text{ g}$$

The total weight of the suppository mixture is:

menthol	0.6 g
paracetamol	3.6 g
theobroma base	8.74 g
total weight	12.94 g

therefore each individual suppository will weigh 1.08 g.

Glyco gelatin suppository bases

Glyco gelatin bases provide an aqueous base for the preparation of suppositories or pessaries. Again the drug can be incorporated into the base and if a specified quantity per suppository is prescribed, then the displacement value of the drug must be used in calculating the amount of base required.

The glyco gelatin base is denser than the theobroma oil or the waxy type bases. It is estimated that 1.2 g of glyco gelatin base occupies the same volume as 1 g of theobroma oil. When calculating the amount of glyco gelatin base required, it is important to take this factor into account. Thus, a nominal 1 g mould will hold 1.2 g of glyco gelatin base, and a 2 g mould will hold 2.4 g.

EXAMPLE 7.8

A pharmacist has to prepare twenty 2 g glyco gelatin pessaries each containing 150 mg miconazole nitrate. The displacement value of miconazole nitrate is 1.6. Assuming that for ease of preparation that the pharmacist makes sufficient for 25 pessaries, calculate the weight of miconazole nitrate and glyco gelatin base required for the preparation of 25 pessaries.

First calculate the displacement due to the drug. 25 pessaries will contain 3750 mg (25 pessaries × 150 mg of miconazole nitrate).
Converting milligrams to grams:

$$
\begin{array}{ccccc}
 & g & - & - & mg \\
3750\ mg = & 3 & 7 & 5 & 0 \quad = 3.75\ g
\end{array}
$$

Let the displacement due to the drug be y. Setting up proportional sets:

mass of miconazole (g)	1.6	3.75
base displaced (g)	1	y

$$\frac{y}{3.75} = \frac{1}{1.6}$$

$$y = 2.344$$

3.75 g of miconazole nitrate is required for 25 pessaries and this quantity of drug will displace 2.344 g of base. However, the displacement value is determined for a theobroma oil type base not a glyco gelatin base. If 25 theobroma oil pessaries were to be produced then the amount of base required would be:

$(25 \text{ pessaries} \times 2 \text{ g}) - 2.344 \text{ g}$ (quantity displaced by the drug)

Since the 1.2 g of the glyco gelatin base is equal to 1 g of the theobroma oil base, then the amount of glyco gelatin base required is:

$1.2 \, [(25 \times 2) - 2.344] = 57.19 \text{ g of glyco gelatin base}$

The final formula for the pessaries is:

miconazole nitrate	3.75 g
glyco gelatin base	57.19 g
total weight	60.94 g

therefore each nominal 2 g pessary will weigh 2.44 g.

......

The difference between the nominal weight of the pessary and the actual weight is mainly due to the weight of the glyco gelatin base.

Note: If the quantity of drug to be incorporated into a suppository or pessary is expressed as a percentage then it is not necessary to use a displacement value.

EXAMPLE 7.9

A pharmacist has to prepare 20 g of suppository mixture to the formula:

zinc oxide	*10%*
calamine	*15%*
suppository base to	*100%*

Calculate the required quantities of each ingredient in the formula.

In this situation the quantities will be calculated in the usual way.

Let the required quantities of zinc oxide and calamine, respectively, be x and y. Setting up proportional sets:

	amount (g)	percentage
zinc oxide	x	10
calamine	y	15
suppository base	20	100

We can spot that 100 is divided by 5 to give 20, so 15 is divided by 5 to give y and 10 is divided by 5 to give x, therefore:

$x = 2$

$y = 3$

The formula for 20 g of suppository mixture is:

zinc oxide	2 g
calamine	3 g
suppository base to	20 g (i.e. 20 – 2 – 3 = 15 g)

Density

The density of a liquid is the weight per unit volume and is expressed as grams per millilitre. This value can be used to convert a volume to a weight or vice versa. The conversion to a weight or volume may in practice be for the convenience of the formulator. For example, in the case of a very mobile liquid it may be easier to measure by volume rather than have to weigh the liquid. Alternatively, if the liquid is very viscous, it may be easier to convert a volume to a weight and weigh the viscous liquid. In Example 7.10 a volume is converted to a weight.

EXAMPLE 7.10

Using a weight per millilitre of 0.98 g, convert 15 mL of liquid X to its equivalent weight.

Let the weight of 15 mL of liquid X be y. Setting up proportional sets:

mass (g)	0.98	y
volume (mL)	1	15

$$\frac{y}{15} = \frac{0.98}{1}$$

$$y = 14.7$$

15 mL of liquid X has a mass of 14.7 g.

In Example 7.11 a weight is converted into a volume.

EXAMPLE 7.11

Using a weight per millilitre of 1.4 g, convert 34 g of liquid Z to its equivalent volume in millilitres.

Let the volume of liquid Z be *a*. Setting up proportional sets:

mass (g)   1.4   34

volume (mL)   1   *a*

$$\frac{a}{34} = \frac{1}{1.4}$$

$$a = 24.29$$

34 g of liquid Z has a volume of 24.29 mL.

The ability to use density values is needed when a liquid (expressed as a volume) is one of the components of an ointment, cream or gel and the final quantity of the ointment, cream or gel is expressed as a weight.

EXAMPLE 7.12

A pharmacist has to prepare 25 g of an ointment to the following formula:

zinc oxide   *10 g*

liquid paraffin   *15 mL*

yellow soft paraffin to   *100 g*

Calculate the final formula for 25 g of the ointment.

First calculate the quantities for 25 g.

Let the required weight of zinc oxide be x and let the required volume of liquid paraffin be y. Setting up proportional sets:

mass of zinc oxide (g)	10	x
volume of liquid paraffin (mL)	15	y
mass of yellow soft paraffin (g) to	100	25

We can spot that the values in the second column are $\frac{1}{4}$ of those in the first column, therefore:

$x = 2.5$

$y = 3.75$

The quantities for 25 g can be written as:

zinc oxide	2.5 g
liquid paraffin	3.75 mL
yellow soft paraffin to	25 g

From this formula it can be seen that yellow soft paraffin is expressed as a weight. In order to complete the calculation the volume of liquid paraffin will need to be converted into a weight because it is not possible to take 3.75 mL from 25 g (because there are two different units involved, i.e. millilitres and grams). Because the density of liquid paraffin is not 1, then 3.75 mL will not be equivalent to 3.75 g and so 3.75 mL must be converted into an equivalent weight.

The density of liquid paraffin is 0.88 g per millilitre. Let the weight of liquid paraffin be z. Setting up proportional sets:

mass of liquid paraffin (g)	z	0.88
volume of liquid paraffin (mL)	3.75	1

$$\frac{z}{3.75} = \frac{0.88}{1}$$

$z = 3.30$

3.75 mL of liquid paraffin weighs 3.30 g, so the weight of yellow soft paraffin required in the formula is:

$$25 - (3.30 + 2.5) = 19.2 \text{ g}$$

Practice calculations

Answers are given at the end of the chapter.

Q1 Drug Z has a negligible displacement volume in water. If 10 mL of water is added to 50 mg of drug Z, what will be the final volume of the solution?

Q2 A pharmacist adds 75 mL of water to 35 g of a soluble drug powder and the volume of the final solution is 115 mL. Calculate the displacement volume of the drug powder.

Q3 Ampicillin powder for reconstitution into an injection has a displacement volume of 0.8 mL per gram. If 10 mL of water is added to 500 mg of the powder, calculate the total volume of the solution. What is the concentration expressed as mg/mL?

Q4 A prescriber requires an injection solution containing 50 mg vancomycin in 1 mL. 500 mg of vancomycin powder for reconstitution into an injection is available in a vial. The displacement volume for the powder is 0.3 mL per 500 mg. What volume of sterile diluent should be added to the vancomycin powder to produce the required concentration? What is the total volume of the final injection solution?

Q5 Drug X has a displacement volume of 0.1 mL/30 units and is required as an injection containing 6 units in 1 mL. Drug X is available as a powder suitable for reconstitution into an injection in a vial containing 90 units. What volume of diluent should be added to the powder to produce the injection solution?

Q6 A drug is required in the concentration 20 mg/mL. Drug powder suitable for preparing the solution is available with a displacement volume of 0.15 mL/100 mg. How much diluent and how much powder should be used to produce 5 mL of a solution of the required concentration?

The following displacement values may be required for questions 7–13.

aspirin	1.1
camphor	0.7
castor oil	1.0
hydrocortisone	1.5
bismuth subgallate	2.7
sulphur	1.6
zinc sulphate	2.4

Q7 Calculate the quantities required to produce 100 suppositories to the following formula:

> castor oil   10 mg
> zinc sulphate   200 mg
> theobroma oil sufficient to produce a 1 g suppository

Q8 Calculate the quantities required to produce 20 pessaries to the following formula:

> hydrocortisone 150 mg
> waxy pessary base sufficient to produce a 2 g pessary

Assume the pessary base has the same physical characteristics as theobroma oil.

Q9 12 nominal 1 g suppositories each containing 100 mg of camphor and 75 mg of aspirin are prescribed for a patient. Calculate the quantities required if the suppository base is theobroma oil. Assume no excess mixture is prepared.

Q10 Repeat question 9 assuming the suppository base is glyco gelatin. What is the weight of each suppository?

Q11 2 g suppositories each containing 125 mg of bismuth subgallate and 50 mg of sulphur in theobroma oil are required to fill a private prescription. Calculate the quantities required of each component to produce 25 suppositories. What is the weight of each suppository?

Q12 A pharmacist has to make a batch of one hundred 1 g supposi- tories, each containing 75 mg of drug J. Drug J has a displace- ment value of 2.1. Assuming the pharmacist makes a 20% excess to allow for losses in preparation and the base is glyco gelatin, calculate the quantities of base and drug J required. What is the final weight of each suppository?

Q13 A prescription reads:

> Cocaine hydrochloride   10%
> Theobroma oil to   100%
> Send six 1 g suppositories.

Assume the pharmacist needs to make two additional supposi- tories to those prescribed because of the method of preparation. Calculate the quantities required to make the suppository mix.

Q14 Methyl salicylate has a density of 1.18 g/mL. Calculate the weight of 45 mL of methyl salicylate and calculate the volume occupied by 60 g of methyl salicylate.

Q15 25 g of arachis oil is to be incorporated into 250 g of ointment base. If the weight per millilitre of arachis oil is 0.917 g, how many millilitres of arachis oil are equivalent to 25 g?

Q16 Liquid paraffin has a density of 0.91 g/mL. What is the weight of 2 L?. Express your answer in grams and kilograms.

Q17 A pharmacist is required to provide 75 mL of glycerol. A suit- able measure is not available. What weight of glycerol is equival- ent to 75 mL? Assume the density of glycerol is 1.25 g/mL.

Q18 If the weight of 40 mL of a liquid is 37.5 g, what is the density of the liquid in g/mL?

Q19 A prescription states:

> Glycerol   10 mL
> Drug Z   25 g
> Ointment base to   100 g

If the density of glycerol is 1.25 g/mL, give the quantities (in grams) of all the ingredients if 60 g of the ointment is required.

Answers

A1   10 mL

A2   1.14 mL/g

A3   10.4 mL
         48.1 mg/mL

A4   9.7 mL
         10 mL

A5   14.7 mL

A6   4.85 mL
         100 mg

A7   castor oil   1 g
         zinc sulphate   20 g
         theobroma oil $100 - (1 + 8.33) = 90.67$ g

A8   hydrocortisone   3 g
         base $40 - \left(\dfrac{3}{1.5}\right) = 38$ g

A9   camphor   1.2 g
         aspirin   0.9 g
         base $12 - \left(\dfrac{1.2}{0.7} + \dfrac{0.9}{1.1}\right) = 12 - (1.71 + 0.82) = 9.47$ g

A10   glyco gelatin base = $9.47 \times 1.2 = 11.36$
         base plus ingredients = $11.36 + 1.2 + 0.9 = 13.46$
         each suppository = 1.12 g

A11

	for 1 suppository	for 25 suppositories
bismuth subgallate	125 mg	3.125 g
sulphur	50 mg	1.25 mg
base to	2 g	$50 - \left(\dfrac{3.125}{2.7} + \dfrac{1.25}{1.6}\right)$
		$= 50 - (1.157 + 0.781)$
		$= 48.06$ g

Weight of each suppository =

$$\frac{48.06 + 3.125 + 1.25}{25} = \frac{52.437}{25} = 2.097 \text{ g}$$

A12

	for one suppository	for 120 suppositories
drug J	75 mg	9 g
base to	1 g	$120 - \left(\frac{9}{2.1}\right) = 115.71 \text{ g}$

If the base is glyco gelatin the required amount is $1.2 \times 115.71 = 138.85$ g.

Weight of each suppository = $\frac{(138.85 + 9)}{120} = 1.232$ g

A13 Sufficient mixture for eight suppositories will be made, i.e. 8 g.
cocaine hydrochloride = 0.8 g
theobroma oil = 7.2 g

A14 53.1 g
50.85 mL

A15 27.26 mL

A16 1820 g = 1.82 kg

A17 93.75 g

A18 0.938 g/mL

A19

glycerol	7.5 g
drug Z	15 g
ointment base	37.5 g

8

Calculations involving molecular weights

Molecular weights of drugs

The molecular weight of a drug is the sum of all the atomic weights of the individual atoms in the molecule expressed in grams. For example, a molecule of sodium chloride (NaCl) consists of one atom of sodium and one atom of chlorine (atomic weights are given in the Appendix), so the molecular weight of sodium chloride is:

Na + Cl

$23 + 35.5 = 58.5$ g

If there is more than one atom of the same kind in a molecule, all the individual atoms must be included in the calculation. For example, aluminium chloride ($AlCl_3$) consists of one atom of aluminium and three atoms of chlorine, so the molecular weight of aluminium chloride is:

$Al + Cl_3$

$27 + (35.5 \times 3) = 133.5$ g

If a molecule has associated water molecules, these must be included in the calculation of molecular weight. For example, the molecular weight of ferrous sulphate ($FeSO_4.7H_2O$) is:

$Fe + S + O_4 + 7(H_2O)$

$56 + 32 + (16 \times 4) + 7 \times [(1 \times 2) + 16] = 278$ g

The formulae of the above molecules are simple. Many drug molecules have much more complicated formulae and to calculate the molecular weight it is easier to use the empirical formula rather than the structural formula. For example, the empirical formula of aspirin is $C_9H_8O_4$, thus the molecular weight can be calculated as follows:

$$(9 \times 12) + (8 \times 1) + (4 \times 16) = 180 \text{ g}$$

The structural formula of aspirin is:

From the structural formula it is not readily clear how many atoms of each element are present. In order to calculate the molecular weight from the structural formula, it is therefore necessary to first determine the empirical formula. However, during the process of converting the structural formula into the empirical formula, it is easy to introduce errors, therefore, wherever possible, if the empirical formula is available it should be used.

Empirical and structural formulae of drugs can be found in official publications, for example *The Pharmaceutical Codex*, *Martindale* and the pharmacopoeias.

Knowledge of the molecular weight of a compound or drug allows the calculation of the amount of a certain element present in that compound or drug.

EXAMPLE 8.1

How many milligrams of fluoride ions are contained in 100 mg of sodium fluoride?

First the atomic weights need to be found for each of the elements and then the molecular weight can be calculated

Na + F

23 + 19 = 42

The molecular weight of sodium fluoride is therefore 42 g and thus the fluoride ion represents 19 parts out of 42 parts of the sodium fluoride molecule.

Let the number of milligrams of fluoride ions in 100 mg of sodium fluoride be x. Setting up proportional sets:

	sodium fluoride	fluoride
mass (mg)	100	x
molecular/atomic weight	42	19

$$\frac{100}{42} = \frac{x}{19}$$

$$x = 45.24$$

100 mg of sodium fluoride contains 45.24 mg of fluoride ions.

Some pharmaceutical calculations require the percentage of a specific component of a drug to be determined. In such cases it may be necessary to use a knowledge of molecular weights.

EXAMPLE 8.2

What is the percentage of lithium contained in 250 mg of lithium carbonate?

First the molecular weight of lithium carbonate must be calculated from the empirical formula and the relevant atomic weights.

$$Li_2 + C + O_3$$

$$(7 \times 2) + 12 + (16 \times 3) = 74$$

The molecular weight of lithium carbonate is 74 g. The lithium represents 14 parts of the 74 parts of the lithium carbonate molecule.

Let the number of milligrams of lithium in 250 mg of lithium carbonate be y. Setting up proportional sets:

	lithium	lithium carbonate
amount (mg)	y	250
molecular/atomic weight	14	74

$$\frac{y}{14} = \frac{250}{74}$$

$$y = 47.30$$

250 mg of lithium carbonate contains 47.3 mg lithium. This can be expressed as a percentage:

$$\frac{47.30}{250} \times 100$$

$$= 18.92\%$$

Alternatively, the percentage of lithium in lithium carbonate can be calculated directly from the ratio of lithium to lithium carbonate using the atomic weights, i.e. by-passing the step involving the calculation of the amount of lithium in lithium carbonate.

Let the required percentage be x. Setting up proportional sets:

	lithium	*lithium carbonate*
percentage	x	100
molecular/atomic weight	14	74

$$\frac{x}{14} = \frac{100}{74}$$

$$x = 18.92$$

There is 18.92% of lithium in 250 mg of lithium carbonate.

Drugs and their salts

Some drugs may be prepared with different salts attached to the basic drug molecule. For example, iron is presented as a number of different ferrous salts. The ferrous salts that are available for use as drugs are fumarate, gluconate, succinate, sulphate and dried sulphate. Although different salts of a drug may be prescribed, it is normal to give an equivalent amount of the base drug. It may therefore be necessary to calculate the equivalent amount of base drug in two different salts.

Equivalent amounts of drug in different salts of that drug

In Example 8.3 we compare two salts of iron in terms of the iron content.

EXAMPLE 8.3
___

What is the iron content in a tablet containing 200 mg of ferrous sulphate (dried) and what weight of ferrous gluconate contains the same quantity of iron?

First let us calculate the molecular weight of ferrous sulphate:

$$Fe + S + O_4$$

$$56 + 32 + (16 \times 4) = 152$$

The molecular weight of ferrous sulphate is 152.

From the above, it can be seen that the iron represents 56 parts of the total 152.

Let the amount of iron in 200 mg of ferrous sulphate be y. Setting up proportional sets:

	iron	*ferrous sulphate*
amount (mg)	y	200
molecular/atomic weight	56	152

$$\frac{y}{56} = \frac{200}{152}$$

$$y = 73.68$$

200 mg of ferrous sulphate contains 73.68 mg of iron.

Now let us tackle the second part of the problem, namely how much ferrous gluconate contains the same amount of elemental iron as 200 mg of ferrous sulphate.

Ferrous gluconate has an empirical formula of $C_{12}H_{22}FeO_{12}.2H_2O$ and a molecular weight of 482. If we look at the empirical formula we can see that it contains one atom of iron, therefore 56 parts of the molecular weight of ferrous gluconate are accounted for by the iron (assuming the atomic weight of the iron equals 56). The problem is to calculate how much ferrous gluconate will contain 73.68 mg of iron.

Let the amount of ferrous gluconate be z. Setting up proportional sets:

amount of iron (mg)	z	73.68
molecular atomic weight	482	56

$z = 634.17$

634.17 mg of ferrous gluconate contains the same amount of iron as 200 mg of ferrous sulphate.

Calculating the weight of the salt, if the drug is expressed as the base

Many drug preparations consist of the salt (or salts) of a base drug. However, in describing the drug preparation it is usual to express the dose or strength in terms of the base drug rather than the actual salt used in the preparation. One such example is the drug clindamycin. The available formulations of clindamycin are as follows:

- the capsules each contain 75 mg clindamycin (as the hydrochloride)
- the paediatric suspension contains 75 mg clindamycin (as the palmitate hydrochloride) per 5 mL
- the injection contains 150 mg clindamycin (as phosphate) per 1 mL.

In other words, the capsules contain an amount of clindamycin hydrochloride that is equivalent to 75 mg of clindamycin and, similarly, the paediatric suspension contains an amount of clindamycin palmitate hydrochloride that is equivalent to 75 mg of clindamycin in every 5 mL. The injection contains the equivalent of 150 mg of clindamycin presented as the phosphate per 1 mL.

If the empirical formulae of clindamycin hydrochloride, clindamycin palmitate hydrochloride and clindamycin phosphate are known, it is possible to calculate the amount of the clindamycin salt required in each preparation, i.e. to give a known quantity of clindamycin.

The molecular weights are:

clindamycin	425
clindamycin hydrochloride	461
clindamycin palmitate hydrochloride	700
clindamycin phosphate	505

EXAMPLE 8.4

Using the above data calculate the amounts of clindamycin hydrochloride (in the capsules) and clindamycin palmitate hydrochloride (in the suspension) that are equivalent to 75 mg clindamycin.

Let the amount of clindamycin hydrochloride be x and the amount of clindamycin palmitate hydrochloride be y. Setting up proportional sets:

	amount (mg)	molecular weight
clindamycin	75	425
clindamycin hydrochloride	x	461
clindamycin palmitate hydrochloride	y	700

$$\frac{x}{75} = \frac{461}{425}$$

and

$$\frac{y}{75} = \frac{700}{425}$$

therefore $x = 81.35$ and $y = 123.53$.

Each capsule will contain 81.35 mg of clindamycin hydrochloride and each 5 mL spoonful of paediatric suspension will contain 123.53 mg of clindamycin palmitate hydrochloride.

Using the same approach the amount of clindamycin in the injection solution can be determined.

EXAMPLE 8.5

Calculate the amount of clindamycin phosphate required in each milli-litre of the injection.

Let the amount of clindamycin phosphate be z. (Remember that each millilitre of injection contains 150 mg of clindamycin (as phosphate)). Setting up proportional sets:

	amount (mg)	molecular weight
clindamycin phosphate	z	505
clindamycin	150	425

$z = 178.24$

Each millilitre of injection contains 178.24 mg of clindamycin phosphate, which is equivalent to 150 mg clindamycin.

Using weights of salts expressed as equivalent to a known weight of base

In some official publications the salts of a drug are expressed as an amount equivalent to a known amount of the anhydrous base. For example, the BNF notes that 'quinine (anhydrous base) 100 mg is equivalent to quinine bisulphate 169 mg is equivalent to quinine dihydrochloride 122 mg', and so on.

EXAMPLE 8.6

Find the relationship between quinine (anhydrous base), quinine bisulphate and quinine dihydrochloride using the proportional sets approach and the molecular weights of the base and its two salts.

The molecular weights are 324, 548 and 397, respectively, for the anhydrous base, bisulphate and dihydrochloride of quinine. Setting up proportional sets:

	equivalents	molecular weight
quinine anhydrous base	100	324
quinine bisulphate	169	548
quinine dihydrochloride	122	397

If the BNF equivalent figures are correct, then each of the above ratios of amount to molecular weight should give the same value.
Calculating each ratio gives:

quinine anhydrous base	0.3086
quinine bisulphate	0.3084
quinine dihydrochloride	0.3073

These ratios are similar and therefore the BNF equivalents are correct.

The equivalent values for the quinine salts can be used to determine the amount of quinine anhydrous base in a tablet containing a quinine salt.

EXAMPLE 8.7

Calculate the amount of quinine base in a quinine bisulphate 300 mg tablet.

Use the equivalent values found in Example 8.6. Let the amount of quinine anhydrous base in a quinine bisulphate 300 mg tablet be x. Setting up proportional sets:

	equivalents	amount (mg)
quinine anhydrous base	100	x
quinine bisulphate	169	300

$$\frac{100}{169} = \frac{x}{300}$$

$$x = 178$$

A quinine bisulphate 300 mg tablet contains 178 mg of quinine anhydrous base.

Drugs and their hydrates

As described above, ferrous sulphate exists in the anhydrous form and as a hydrate. Thus, it will be clear that the same weight of the anhydrous and the hydrate of ferrous sulphate will contain different amounts of iron. In order to calculate the equivalent amounts of iron, it is necessary to take into account the water of hydration in the molecule.

EXAMPLE 8.8

1 L of Paediatric Ferrous Sulphate Oral Solution BP contains 12 g of ferrous sulphate. A pharmacist is required to make 150 mL of this solution, but only ferrous sulphate anhydrous is available. How much ferrous sulphate anhydrous should be used?

First we need to calculate how much ferrous sulphate is required to make 150 mL of the preparation.

Let the required amount of ferrous sulphate be x. (Remember that 1 L equals 1000 mL.) Setting up proportional sets:

| amount of ferrous sulphate (g) | x | 12 |
| volume of solution (mL) | 150 | 1000 |

$$\frac{x}{150} = \frac{12}{1000}$$

$$x = 1.8$$

1.8 g of ferrous sulphate is required to make 150 mL of paediatric solution.

As shown previously, the molecular weights of ferrous sulphate and ferrous sulphate anhydrous are 278 and 152, respectively.

Let the required amount of ferrous sulphate anhydrous be y. Setting up proportional sets:

	amount (g)	*molecular weight*
ferrous sulphate	1.8	278
ferrous sulphate anhydrous	y	152

$$\frac{y}{1.8} = \frac{152}{278}$$

$$y = 0.984$$

0.984 g of ferrous sulphate anhydrous is equivalent to 1.8 g of ferrous sulphate, therefore the pharmacist should use 0.984 g of the anhydrous ferrous sulphate in preparing 150 mL of solution.

....

Another example in which a drug is available in different hydrated forms is codeine phosphate. The *British Pharmacopoeia* directs that 30 mg codeine phosphate tablets contain codeine phosphate or the equivalent amount of codeine phosphate sesquihydrate.

EXAMPLE 8.9

How much codeine phosphate sesquihydrate is equivalent to 30 mg of codeine phosphate?

If we look at the formulae for both phosphates, it can be seen that Codeine Phosphate BP exists as the hemihydrate and has a molecular weight of 406 and that codeine sesquihydrate has a molecular weight of 424. The difference in the molecular weights is due to one molecule of water, i.e. the difference between a sesqui and a hemi hydrate. We can calculate the amount of codeine phosphate sesquihydrate equivalent to 30 mg of codeine phosphate.

Let the amount of codeine phosphate sesquihydrate be z. Setting up proportional sets:

	amount (mg)	molecular weight
codeine phosphate hemihydrate	30	406
codeine phosphate sesquihydrate	z	424

$$\frac{z}{30} = \frac{424}{406}$$

$z = 31.33$

A 30 mg codeine phosphate tablet would contain 30 mg of codeine phosphate hemihydrate or 31.33 mg codeine phosphate sesquihydrate.

....

Calculation of legal classifications using molecular weights

If a drug is available as different salts, then the legal classification of each salt may be based on the equivalent amount of base drug. In the UK, examples of such drugs are pholcodine and its salts, morphine and its salts, hyoscyamine hydrobromide and sulphate, ephedrine hydrochloride and quinine and its salts.

Classification based on maximum dose (calculated as base)

Lithium carbonate is a prescription-only medicine, but if it is in a preparation intended for internal use with a maximum dose of 5 mg (calculated as base) and a maximum daily dose of 15 mg (calculated as base) the preparation can be sold over the counter (*Medicines, Ethics and Practice*, issue 24, July 2000). Therefore, in order to ascertain the legal classification of a lithium carbonate preparation it is necessary to calculate the equivalent amount of lithium base.

EXAMPLE 8.10

What is the maximum dose and daily dose of lithium carbonate that can be sold over the counter?

The molecular weight of lithium carbonate is 74 and the molecular weight of lithium is 14.

Let the maximum dose of lithium carbonate be x and the maximum daily dose of lithium carbonate be y. Setting up proportional sets:

	lithium	lithium carbonate
molecular/atomic weights	14	74
maximum dose (mg)	5	x
maximum daily dose (mg)	15	y

$$\frac{14}{74} = \frac{15}{x}$$

and

$$\frac{14}{74} = \frac{15}{y}$$

therefore

$$x = 26.43 \text{ and } y = 79.29$$

A preparation of lithium carbonate can be sold over the counter provided that it has a maximum dose of 26.43 mg and a maximum daily dose of 79.29 mg. If either one or both of these doses are exceeded then the preparation becomes a prescription-only medicine.

Classification based on maximum strength of base

In some legal classifications, the maximum dose is not stipulated but a maximum strength is stated. For example, morphine and its salts are Schedule 2 Controlled Drugs, but in the case of the salts, if the morphine cannot be readily recovered and in liquid preparations with a maximum strength of 0.2% (calculated as the anhydrous morphine base) the preparation becomes a Schedule 5 Controlled Drug.

In order to determine the legal classification of liquid preparations of morphine salts, it is therefore necessary to calculate the weight of the anhydrous morphine base.

EXAMPLE 8.11

What is the maximum amount of morphine sulphate that can be incorporated into 200 mL of a liquid preparation so that the legal classification is a Schedule 5 Controlled Drug?

The molecular weights of anhydrous morphine base and morphine sulphate are 285 and 759, respectively. A 0.2% solution will contain 0.2 g in 100 mL and therefore 0.4 g in 200 mL. The equivalent of 0.4 g of anhydrous base (in the form of morphine sulphate) is the maximum amount allowed in the liquid preparation, if it is to be classified as a Schedule 5 Controlled Drug.

Let the amount of morphine sulphate be x. Setting up proportional sets:

	amount (g)	molecular weight
morphine sulphate	x	759
morphine anhydrous base	0.4	285

$$\frac{759}{285} = \frac{x}{0.4}$$

$$x = 1.065$$

1.065 g of morphine sulphate is equivalent to 0.4 g of anhydrous morphine base. The maximum amount of morphine sulphate that can be incorporated into 200 mL of a liquid preparation so that the legal classification is Schedule 5 Controlled Drug is 1.065 g.

Classification based on maximum strength and maximum dose

Some legal classifications are based on a maximum strength and a maximum dose, for example codeine. The *Medicines, Ethics and Practice* guide states that 'In single dose preparations with a maximum strength per dosage unit of 1.5% (calculated as base) and a maximum dose of 20 mg (calculated as base) codeine and its salts are classified as Schedule 5 Controlled Drug medicines'.

EXAMPLE 8.12

A capsule containing codeine sulphate has a recommended dose of 20 mg (calculated as base). What is the weight of the codeine sulphate and the maximum weight of the capsule contents that will mean it should be classified as a Schedule 5 Controlled Drug medicine?

First it is necessary to calculate the weight of codeine sulphate equivalent to 20 mg of codeine base:

codeine base has a molecular weight of 317 g

codeine sulphate has a molecular weight of 750 g

Let the weight of codeine sulphate be x. Setting up proportional sets:

	amount (mg)	molecular weight
codeine sulphate	x	750
codeine base	20	317

$$\frac{x}{20} = \frac{750}{317}$$

$x = 47.32$

The capsule will contain 47.32 mg of codeine sulphate.

For the capsule to be a Schedule 5 Controlled Drug, the codeine sulphate (calculated as base) must not be more than 1.5% of the overall weight of the capsule. (Remember that a capsule will contain excipients, such as starch, as well as the drug.)

If 20 mg of base is equal to 1.5%, i.e. 1.5/100, then let the overall weight in milligrams be y. Setting up proportional sets:

amount of codeine phosphate (mg)   20   1.5

overall weight (mg) y 100

$$\frac{100}{1.5} = \frac{y}{20}$$

$$y = 1333$$

Converting this to grams gives 1.333 g, therefore the overall weight of the capsule contents should not be less than 1.333 g if the preparation is to be classified as a Schedule 5 Controlled Drug.

Moles and millimoles

The atomic and molecular weights of a drug or excipient can be used as a method of defining an amount of a drug or excipient. In this method, the term *mole* is used. The mole is the SI base unit for the amount of a substance. The substance can be atoms, molecules or ions, and the mole is the atomic, molecular or ionic weight expressed in grams. For example, the atomic weight of iron is 56 and so 1 mole of iron weighs 56 g. Similarly, the molecular weight of sodium chloride is 58.5 g (see previously), therefore a mole of sodium chloride weighs 58.5 g and 2 moles of sodium chloride weighs $58.5 \times 2 = 117$ g.

However, a molecule of sodium chloride consists of one sodium ion and one chloride ion. Since moles can refer to ions as well as molecules, it can be seen that one mole of sodium chloride contains one mole of sodium and one mole of chloride, therefore:

1 mole of sodium chloride weighs 58.5 g

1 mole of sodium ion weighs 23 g

1 mole of chloride ion weighs 35.5 g

Now consider ferrous sulphate, $FeSO_4.7H_2O$. The molecular weight is 278 and so 1 mole weighs 278 g. However, from the molecular formula and a knowledge of the atomic weights it can be seen that ferrous sulphate contains:

1 mole of Fe = 56 g

1 mole of S = 32 g

4 moles of O, each mole of O = 16 g

7 moles of H_2O, each mole of water = 18 g.

In the same way that the system of weights and volumes have multiples and subdivisions (milli, micro, nano, etc.), so the mole has similar subdivisions and multiples:

1 mole contains 1000 millimoles (mmol)

1 millimole contains 1000 micromoles

1 micromole contains 1000 nanomoles

1 nanomole contains 1000 picomoles

Again we can use a place value approach:

moles – – millimoles – – micromoles – – nanomoles

Using these column headings it can be seen that 2 millimoles is equivalent to 0.002 moles or 2000 micromoles or 2 000 000 nanomoles:

moles	–	–	millimoles	–	–	micromoles	–	–	nanomoles
			2	0	0	0	0	0	0

Similarly, 15 micromoles is equivalent to 0.015 millimoles or 15 000 nanomoles:

millimoles	–	–	micromoles	–	–	nanomoles
	1	5	0	0	0	

Because moles are relatively large quantities (for example 1 mole of clindamycin is 425 g), the subdivisions of the mole are frequently used for pharmaceuticals.

The quantities of many drugs, especially electrolytes, are expressed in moles or their subdivisions.

EXAMPLE 8.13

The BNF states that sodium bicarbonate capsules each contain 500 mg sodium bicarbonate (approximately 6 millimoles each of Na⁺ and HCO³⁻). Verify this statement.

In order to confirm the number of millimoles, it is necessary to consider the molecular formula of sodium bicarbonate. Sodium bicarbonate consists of one ion of sodium and one ion of bicarbonate:

$$NaHCO_3 = Na^+ + HCO^{3-}$$

1 mole of sodium bicarbonate weighs 84 g and contains 1 mole of sodium and 1 mole of bicarbonate ion.

The relationship between mass of drug and number of moles is proportional, therefore for sodium bicarbonate capsules each weighing 500 mg, let the number of moles be y. (Remember to keep the units of weight the same, i.e. if the molecular weight is in grams then the weight of the drug should be in grams (500 mg = 0.5 g).) Setting up proportional sets:

number of moles	y	1
amount of sodium bicarbonate (g)	0.5	84

$$\frac{y}{0.5} = \frac{1}{84}$$

$$y = 0.0059$$

A sodium bicarbonate capsule will contain 0.0059 moles (5.9 millimoles) of sodium bicarbonate. Because 1 mole of sodium bicarbonate consists of 1 mole of sodium and 1 mole of bicarbonate, 5.9 millimoles of sodium bicarbonate will contain 5.9 millimoles of sodium and 5.9 millimoles of bicarbonate ion. These values approximate to 6 millimoles, and so we have confirmed the information given in the BNF.

If a molecule contains more than one ion of the same species, then care must be taken in calculating the number of moles.

EXAMPLE 8.14

Calculate the number of moles of chloride ion in 500 mg of calcium chloride.

1 mole of calcium chloride ($CaCl_2$) consists of 1 mole of calcium and 2 moles of chloride ion, therefore in order to calculate the number of moles of chloride ion in 500 mg of calcium chloride, it is necessary to calculate the number of moles of calcium chloride.

Let the number of moles of calcium chloride be z. The molecular weight of calcium chloride is 110 g. (Remember to keep the weights in the same units, i.e. convert 500 mg to 0.5 g.) Setting up proportional sets:

number of moles	z	1
amount of calcium chloride (g)	0.5	110

$$\frac{z}{0.5} = \frac{1}{110}$$

$$z = 0.0045$$

The number of moles of calcium chloride is 0.0045 = 4.5 millimoles, therefore 500 mg calcium chloride contains 4.5 millimoles of calcium chloride. It also contains 4.5 millimoles of calcium and 9.0 millimoles (4.5×2) of chloride ions, since there are twice as many chloride ions as calcium ions in calcium chloride.

If a salt contains water of crystallisation, then this should be taken into account when calculating moles. For example, a hydrated form of calcium chloride is $CaCl_2.6H_2O$. A mole of this hydrated form of calcium chloride will contain 1 mole of calcium ion, 2 moles of chloride ion and 6 moles of water.

EXAMPLE 8.15

Using the above information, calculate the number of moles of water in 500 mg of $CaCl_2.6H_2O$.

The molecular weight of this molecule is 219 and contains 6 moles of water. The number of moles of water in 500 mg (0.5 g) of hydrated calcium chloride can be calculated.

Let the number of moles of water be y. Setting up proportional sets:

number of moles of water $\qquad\qquad\qquad\qquad y \qquad 6$

amount of hydrated calcium chloride (g) $0.5 \quad 219$

$$\frac{y}{0.5} = \frac{6}{219}$$

$y = 0.0137$

There are 0.0137 moles of water = 13.7 millimoles.

Molar solutions

Since a mole of a substance is defined as a weight, moles are one way of expressing a quantity or an amount. If 1 mole of a substance is dissolved in a solvent and the resulting solution made up to 1 L, then we have 1 mole in 1 L, which is an expression of concentration. This concentration can also be written as 1 mol/L or 1 mol.L^{-1}. Traditionally, the concentration of 1 mole per litre is called a *molar* solution.

For example, a 1 molar aqueous solution of sodium chloride is equivalent to 58.5 g of sodium chloride dissolved in sufficient water to produce 1 L of solution. In other words, molarity refers to the number of moles of solute per litre of solution. Since the term 'molar' is a concentration, it is not necessary to always prepare 1 L of the solution; smaller volumes can be prepared.

EXAMPLE 8.16

How many moles of solute are there in 200 mL of a 1 molar solution?

Let the number of moles of solute be y. Setting up proportional sets:

number of moles $\qquad\qquad\qquad\qquad y \qquad 1$

volume of molar solution (mL) $200 \quad 1000$

$$\frac{y}{200} = \frac{1}{1000}$$

$y = 0.2$

There are 0.2 moles of solute in 200 mL of 1 molar solution.

It may be necessary to calculate the mass of a drug required to prepare a solution expressed in molar terms.

EXAMPLE 8.17

How much sodium chloride is required to make 25 mL of a 0.5 molar solution? How many moles of sodium ion will there be in the final solution?

First it is necessary to find the molecular weights of sodium and sodium chloride, and calculate how many moles of each are contained in 25 mL. The molecular weight of sodium is 23 g and that of sodium chloride is 58.5 g.

Let the number of moles of sodium chloride in 25 mL be y. Setting up proportional sets:

| number of moles | y | 0.5 |
| volume of solution (mL) | 25 | 1000 |

$$\frac{y}{25} = \frac{0.5}{1000}$$

$y = 0.0125$

There are 0.0125 moles of sodium chloride in 25 mL.
The mass of sodium chloride that is contained in 0.0125 moles of sodium chloride is obtained from the number of moles (0.0125) times the molecular weight of sodium chloride, that is 0.73125 g of sodium chloride. 0.73 g of sodium chloride would therefore be required to make 25 mL of a 0.5 molar solution. However, we know that 1 mole of sodium chloride contains 1 mole of sodium ions, therefore the solution of sodium chloride will contain the same number of moles of sodium chloride as sodium, i.e. 25 mL of a 0.5 molar solution of sodium chloride will contain 0.0125 moles of sodium ions.

Because the molecular weights of many drugs are large, for example the molecular weights of cortisone, glibenclamide and nifedipine are 402,

494 and 346, respectively, solubility constraints make it impossible to prepare 1 molar solutions. Also, in many instances molar concentrations of drugs are above the required therapeutic level, therefore such drugs are prepared in concentrations such as millimoles/L, millimoles/mL or even picomoles/mL.

EXAMPLE 8.18

How many millimoles of sodium and chloride ions are contained in 1 L of Sodium Chloride Infusion BP? Sodium Chloride Infusion BP contains 0.9% sodium chloride.

We know from Example 8.17 that 1 mole of sodium chloride contains 1 mole of sodium ions and 1 mole of chloride ions, and that the weight of 1 mole of sodium chloride is 58.5 g. We can also calculate that there are 9 g of sodium chloride in 1 L of 0.9% sodium chloride.

Let the number of moles of sodium chloride in 1 L be x. Setting up proportional sets:

number of moles	x	1
mass of sodium chloride (g)	9	58.5

$$\frac{x}{9} = \frac{1}{58.5}$$

$$x = 0.154$$

There are 0.154 moles of sodium chloride in 1 L of Sodium Chloride Infusion BP, so there are also 0.154 moles of sodium ions and 0.154 moles of chloride ions in 1 L of Sodium Chloride Infusion BP. Using the place value approach, it can be seen that 0.154 moles is equal to 154 millimoles. Thus Sodium Chloride Infusion BP contains 154 milli-moles/L of sodium ions and chloride ions.

Some infusion fluids may contain more than one electrolyte, for example Potassium Chloride and Sodium Chloride Infusion Fluid BP. In such fluids the chloride ion concentration will be the sum of the chloride ion concentrations of both the potassium and the sodium salts.

EXAMPLE 8.19

How many millimoles/L of chloride ions are contained in Potassium Chloride and Sodium Chloride Infusion BP?

The infusion fluid contains:

  potassium chloride 0.3%   (3 g in 1 L)

  sodium chloride 0.9%   (9 g in 1 L)

We know from the chemical formulae that 1 mole of both potassium chloride and sodium chloride would each contain 1 mole of chloride ions, therefore in order to calculate the number of moles of chloride ions in the infusion, we need to calculate the number of moles of both the potassium chloride and the sodium chloride. The molecular weights of sodium chloride and potassium chloride are, respectively, 58.5 and 74.5. The number of moles per litre of sodium chloride are calculated in Example 8.18 to be 154 millimoles, so we need to calculate the number of moles of potassium chloride by the same method.

Let the number of moles of potassium chloride in 1 L be x. Setting up proportional sets:

  number of moles of potassium chloride x 1

  amount of potassium chloride (g)   3   74.5

$$\frac{x}{3} = \frac{1}{74.5}$$
$$x = 0.04$$

There are 0.04 moles of potassium chloride in 1 L, therefore the sodium chloride will contribute 0.154 moles of chloride ions to the infusion fluid and the potassium chloride will contribute 0.04 moles of chloride ions. This is a total of 0.194 moles of chloride ions. Converting moles to millimoles will give 194 millimoles of chloride ions in 1 L of infusion fluid.

From the above it can be seen that Potassium Chloride and Sodium Chloride Infusion BP will contain 154 millimoles of sodium ions and 40 millimoles of potassium ions per litre.

Example 8.20 involves calculating the mass of a drug required to prepare a known volume of a solution expressed in moles per litre.

EXAMPLE 8.20

How much sodium fluoride will be required to make 250 mL of a mouthwash containing 0.012 mol/L of sodium fluoride?

The molecular weight of sodium fluoride is 42, therefore a 1 molar solution will contain 42 g in 1 L.

Let the number of grams of sodium fluoride in 0.012 moles be x. Setting up proportional sets:

number of moles	0.012	1
amount of sodium fluoride (g)	x	42

$$\frac{0.012}{x} = \frac{1}{42}$$

$x = 0.504$

0.504 g of sodium fluoride is required to make 1 L of 0.012 mol/L mouthwash.

Let the quantity of sodium fluoride required to make 250 mL of mouthwash be y. Setting up proportional sets:

amount of sodium fluoride (g)	y	0.504
volume of mouthwash (mL)	250	1000

$$\frac{y}{250} = \frac{0.504}{1000}$$

$y = 0.126$

0.126 g of sodium fluoride is required to make 250 mL of mouthwash.

Milliequivalents

If the concentrations of electrolyte solutions are expressed in moles or other units of weight, there is no indication of the number of ions or the charge that they carry. The gram equivalent was developed to address this situation. Because the gram equivalent is usually large, the smaller unit, the milliequivalent (one thousandth of a gram equivalent), is the generally accepted unit.

A gram equivalent is defined as:

$$\frac{\text{atomic weight of an ion}}{\text{valency of that ion}}$$

The gram equivalents of sodium and calcium are:

sodium: $\frac{23}{1}$ calcium: $\frac{40.1}{2}$

i.e.

gram equivalent of sodium = 23

gram equivalent of calcium = 20

or

1 milliequivalent of sodium = 23 mg

1 milliequivalent of calcium = 20 mg

EXAMPLE 8.21

How many milliequivalents of sodium are there in 1 L of 0.9% sodium chloride infusion?

There is 9 g of sodium chloride in 1 L of infusion. The molecular weight in grams of sodium chloride will contain one gram equivalent of sodium ion. The molecular weight of sodium chloride is 58.5.
    Let the number of gram equivalents of sodium ion in 1 L of infusion be y. Setting up proportional sets:

| number of gram equivalents | y | 1 |
| amount of sodium chloride (g) | 9 | 58.5 |

$$\frac{y}{9} = \frac{1}{58.5}$$

$$y = 0.154$$

There are 0.154 gram equivalents of sodium ion in 1 L. Since these gram equivalents are contained in 1 L, there must be 154 milliequivalents of sodium ion in 1 L of infusion fluid.

The use of milliequivalents has largely been superseded by the use of moles and their subdivisions.

Practice calculations

Answers are given at the end of the chapter.

Q1 For the following drugs calculate the molecular weight, the weight of salt containing 1 millimole of the metal ion and the weight of salt containing 1 milliequivalent of metal ion:

(a) potassium chloride, KCl
(b) sodium chloride, $NaCl$
(c) calcium chloride, $CaCl_2.2H_2O$
(d) calcium lactate, $C_6H_{10}CaO_6.5H_2O$
(e) potassium bicarbonate, $KHCO_3$
(f) magnesium chloride, $MgCl_2.6H_2O$
(g) sodium citrate, $C_6H_5Na_3O_7.2H_2O$
(h) ammonium chloride, NH_4Cl.

Q2 (a) Calculate the molecular weight of lithium citrate $(C_6H_5Li_3O_7.H_2O)$.
(b) What is the percentage of Li^+ in lithium citrate?

Q3 (a) The empirical formula of ferrous fumarate is $C_4H_2FeO_4$. Calculate its molecular weight.
(b) Calculate the weight of ferrous fumarate that will give 100 mg of iron.

Q4 A syrup contains ferrous fumarate 140 mg/5 mL. How much iron will a patient receive per day if the daily dosage regimen is 10 mL twice a day?

Q5 A syrup contains 7.5% of potassium chloride. How many millimoles of K^+ are contained in 1 mL of this syrup?

Q6 Glucose intravenous infusion contains 5% glucose expressed as anhydrous glucose.

(a) How much anhydrous glucose (molecular weight = 180) will be required to prepare 500 mL?

(b)   How much glucose monohydrate (molecular weight = 192) will be required to produce 750 mL of the infusion?

Q7   Calcium gluconate (molecular weight 448.4) tablets each contain 53.4 mg of calcium.

(a)   How much calcium gluconate does each tablet contain?
(b)   How many millimoles of calcium are there in each tablet?

Q8   (a)   What is the molecular weight of calcium acetate ($C_4H_6CaO_4$)?
(b)   Calculate the amount of calcium provided by 300 mg of calcium acetate.
(c)   How many milligrams of calcium acetate are there in 1 millimole?
(d)   How many milligrams of calcium acetate would contain 1 milliequivalent of calcium ion?

Q9   (a)   What is the molecular weight of calcium phosphate ($Ca_3(PO_4)_2$)?
(b)   A powder contains 3.3 g of calcium phosphate. How many millimoles of calcium ion are provided by each powder?

Q10   Magnesium sulphate injection is 50% magnesium sulphate ($MgSO_4.7H_2O$). How many millimoles of magnesium ion per millilitre does the injection contain?

Q11   Sodium Fluoride BP drops contain 275 micrograms of sodium fluoride per drop. Calculate the quantity of fluoride ion provided by five drops of this preparation.

Q12   Ranitidine Injection BP contains ranitidine 25 mg/mL (as the hydrochloride). Calculate the amount of ranitidine hydrochloride needed to prepare 100 mL of injection. (Molecular weights: ranitidine hydrochloride = 350.9, ranitidine = 314.4.)

Q13   The term 'low sodium' indicates a sodium content of less than 1 millimole per tablet or 10 mL dose. What is the maximum amount of sodium chloride that can be contained in a 10 mL dose in order that the preparation can be labelled as 'low sodium'?

Q14 A syrup contains chloroquine sulphate (molecular weight = 436), 68 mg/5 mL dose. Calculate the amount of chloroquine base (molecular weight = 319.9) in each 5 mL dose.

Q15 How much chloroquine base (molecular weight = 319.9) is equivalent to a tablet containing 250 mg chloroquine phosphate (molecular weight = 515.9)?

Q16 How much morphine (molecular weight = 285.3) is contained in 50 mL of a 2% solution of morphine tartrate (molecular weight = 774.8)?

Q17 A patient requires 300 mg of quinine (molecular weight = 324.4). What weight of quinine hydrobromide (molecular weight = 423.3) will provide 300 mg of quinine?

Q18 How much hyoscine (molecular weight = 303.4) is contained in a 20 mg tablet of hyoscine butyl bromide (molecular weight = 440.4)?

Answers

A1

		Molecular weight	Weight of 1 millimole (mg)	Weight of 1 milliequivalent (mg)
	(a)	74.5	74.5	74.5
	(b)	58.5	58.5	58.5
	(c)	147	147	73.5
	(d)	308	308	154
	(e)	100	100	100
	(f)	203	203	101.5
	(g)	294.1	98	98
	(h)	53.5	53.5	53.5

A2 (a) 228
(b) 9.21%

A3 (a) 169.9
(b) 304 mg

A4 184 mg

A5   1 millimole

A6   (a)   25 g
          (b)   40 g

A7   (a)   597.4 mg
          (b)   1.33 millimoles

A8   (a)   158
          (b)   75.9 mg
          (c)   158 mg
          (d)   79 mg

A9   (a)   310
          (b)   32 millimoles

A10   2 millimoles/mL

A11   622 micrograms

A12   2.79 g

A13   58.5 mg

A14   49.9 mg

A15   155 mg

A16   0.368 g

A17   391.5 mg

A18   13.8 mg

9

Parenteral solutions and isotonicity

Many patients receive drugs via the intravenous route, that is directly into a vein. The solution containing the drug is sterile. If the volume to be delivered is a few millilitres or less, the solution (normally termed an injection) is usually administered in one go. If the volume to be delivered is large, it will be administered over a period of time. Such a process is termed intravenous infusion. In order to deliver an intravenous infusion at a constant rate, a 'giving' or administration device consisting of an electrically driven pump is used. The administration pump is set to deliver a chosen number of drops or millilitres per minute or unit of time.

With intravenous infusions, it may be necessary to calculate the volume of solution that is delivered over a period of time or the volume of solution that will deliver a known quantity of drug.

Rate of flow of intravenous solutions

Volume delivered over a specific time period

Calculations involving intravenous infusions may require the determination of the volume of drug solution delivered per period of time. This volume may be expressed as millilitres per minute or hour, or converted to drops per minute.

EXAMPLE 9.1

1000 mL of normal saline solution is to be given to a patient over an 8-hour period. If 20 drops = 1 mL, how many drops per minute should be administered?

The answer needs to be in minutes, so 8 hours is converted to 480 minutes.

The next stage involves calculating the number of drops in 1000 mL. Let the number of drops be x. Setting up proportional sets:

number of drops	x	20
volume of solution (mL)	1000	1

$$\frac{x}{1000} = \frac{20}{1}$$

$$x = 20\,000$$

There are 20 000 drops in 1000 mL.

The infusion (of 20 000 drops) takes 480 minutes to complete. Let the number of drops per minute be y. Setting up proportional sets:

number of drops	20 000	y
number of minutes	480	1

$$\frac{y}{1} = \frac{20\,000}{480}$$

$$y = 41.67$$

The intravenous administration set should be set at 42 drops per minute.

For some intravenous solutions a recommended flow rate is given. In this case, it may be necessary to calculate the overall volume to be delivered and the number of drops per minute.

EXAMPLE 9.2

The recommended flow rate for kanamycin is 3–4 mL per minute at a concentration of 2.5 mg/mL. Kanamycin is supplied in 1 g vials for dilution in glucose 5%. Using a 1 mL vial, what volume of glucose 5% solution should be used and how many drops per minute should be delivered if the flow rate is 4 mL per minute? The intravenous administration set is calibrated to 20 drops per millilitre. How long will the infusion take?

It is necessary to calculate the volume of glucose 5% required to produce a solution containing 2.5 mg of kanamycin per millilitre. A vial of kanamycin contains 1 g, that is 1000 mg.

Let the volume of solution required to contain 2.5 mg/mL be y. Setting up proportional sets:

mass of kanamycin (mg)   2.5   1000

volume of solution (mL)   1 y

$$\frac{y}{1000} = \frac{1}{2.5}$$

$$y = \frac{1000}{2.5}$$

$$y = 400$$

The vial of kanamycin should be dissolved in sufficient glucose 5% to produce 400 mL of solution.

Knowing that the intravenous administration set delivers 20 drops per millilitre, the number of drops in 4 mL can be calculated. Let the number of drops be x. Setting up proportional sets:

number of drops x 20

volume (mL)   4   1

We can spot that 1 is multiplied by 4 to give 4, so 20 is multiplied by 4 to give x, therefore:

$$x = 80$$

A flow rate of 80 drops per minute will deliver 4 mL in one minute.

Let the time taken to administer 400 mL of infusion solution be t. Setting up proportional sets:

time (minutes) t 1

volume (mL)   400   4

We can spot that 4 is multiplied by 100 to give 400, so 1 is multiplied by 100 to give t, therefore:

$$t = 100$$

The time taken to deliver 400 mL is 100 minutes (1 hour 40 minutes).

In some situations, two or more injection solutions may be combined and delivered by intravenous infusion over a known time period. In such cases it is important to remember that the total volume of all the injection solutions should be included in the calculation.

EXAMPLE 9.3

---

10 mL of potassium chloride solution, strong, and 10 mL of multi-vitamin infusion are added to 500 mL of normal saline solution. The resultant solution is to be administered over 4 hours. The administration set is calibrated to 12 drops per millilitre. Calculate the number of drops per minute to be given if the patient is to receive all of the solution in the specified time.

The total volume of the infusion solution is:

10 + 10 + 500 = 520 mL

therefore 520 mL of solution must be infused over 4 hours.

Since we need to calculate the number of drops per minute, we will need to convert the total infusion time to minutes:

total infusion time = 4 × 60 = 240 minutes

The administration set gives 12 drops per millilitre and so we need to convert the total infusion volume into drops. Let the number of drops be x. Setting up proportional sets:

number of drops	12	x
volume (mL)	1	520

We can spot that 1 is multiplied by 520 to give 520, so 12 is multiplied by 520 to give x, therefore:

$x = 6240$

520 mL is equal to 6240 drops.

6240 drops of infusion solution will need to be delivered over 240 minutes. Let the number of drops per minute required to deliver the infusion solution be y. Setting up proportional sets:

number of drops	y	6240
time (minutes)	1	240

$$y = \frac{6240}{240}$$

$$y = 26$$

The infusion fluid should be infused at 26 drops per minute.

Amount of drug delivered over a specified time period

For some drugs, the intravenous administration is stated as the amount of drug, rather than the volume, to be infused over a specified time period.

EXAMPLE 9.4

Phenytoin has a recommended dose of 15 mg per kilogram of body weight to be infused at a rate not exceeding 50 mg per minute. The patient is an adult female weighing 56 kg. Phenytoin injection is available in 5 mL ampoules containing 50 mg/mL. The prescriber would like an infusion volume of 100 mL and a dose rate of 25 mg/minute. Is the prescriber's request possible and if so, what is the flow rate per minute?

It is necessary to calculate the recommended dose for the patient. The patient weighs 56 kg and the dose is 15 mg/kg.

Let the required dose be z. Setting up proportional sets:

dose (mg)	15	z
weight (kg)	1	56

We can spot that 1 is multiplied by 15 to give 15, so 56 is multiplied by 15 to give z, therefore:

$$z = 840$$

The recommended dose for the patient is 840 mg phenytoin.

The injection contains 50 mg/mL. Let the volume of injection be y. Setting up proportional sets:

mass of phenytoin (mg)	840	50
volume of injection (mL)	y	1

We can spot that 50 is divided by 50 to give 1, so 840 is divided by 50 to give y, therefore:

$$y = 16.8$$

16.8 mL of phenytoin injection is required for the recommended dose.

Clearly this volume could be made up to 100 mL with normal saline solution as requested by the prescriber. The resulting 100 mL of solution will contain 840 mg of phenytoin. It is now necessary to calculate the volume per minute that will be needed to deliver 25 mg/minute, i.e. the volume that contains 25 mg of phenytoin.

Let the volume required be x. Setting up proportional sets:

mass of phenytoin (mg)	840	25
volume of solution (mL)	100	x

$$\frac{x}{2.5} = \frac{100}{840}$$

$$x = 2.98$$

2.98 mL contains 25 mg of phenytoin. The flow rate of the infusion should therefore be set at 2.98 mL per minute.

Some drugs are given in much smaller injection volumes through a micropump device. This device enables very small volumes to be delivered at a set rate for a specified time period.

EXAMPLE 9.5

The recommended dose of furosemide (frusemide) by slow intravenous infusion is 50 mg at a rate not exceeding 4 mg per minute. Furosemide injection contains 10 mg furosemide in 1 mL. Calculate the volume of furosemide injection required and the infusion rate, in millilitres per minute, if the patient is to receive the correct dose.

First calculate the volume of injection required. The injection is available as 10 mg/mL and a total of 50 mg is required.

Let the required volume of injection be y. Setting up proportional sets:

volume of injection (mL)	1	y
mass of furosemide (mg)	10	50

We can spot that 10 is multiplied by 5 to give 50, so 1 is multiplied by 5 to give y, therefore:

$y = 5$

5 mL of injection is required and this must be given at a maximum rate of 4 mg/minute. Knowing this maximum rate, we need to calculate the time taken to deliver 50 mg of furosemide at this rate.

Let the time to deliver 50 mg of furosemide be z. Setting up proportional sets:

mass of furosemide (mg)	4	50
time (minutes)	1	z

We can spot that 4 is divided by 4 to give 1, so 50 is divided by 4 to give z, therefore:

$z = 12.5$

It will take 12.5 minutes to deliver all the injection solution at 4 mg/minute.

Let the volume to be delivered in 1 minute be x. Setting up proportional sets:

volume (mL)	5	x
time (minutes)	12.5	1

$$\frac{x}{1} = \frac{5}{12.5}$$

$x = 0.4$

The infusion device should be set at a maximum of 0.4 mL per minute.

··

If a drug is to be administered over a long time period, for example 12 hours or more, then the flow rate may be expressed in milligrams per hour rather than milligrams per minute. In such a case, care must be taken not to confuse minutes with hours, otherwise the dose will be wrong and the treatment of the patient compromised.

EXAMPLE 9.6

A drug is provided as an infusion solution at a concentration of 0.05 mg/mL. The prescribed flow rate is 2 mg per hour. Calculate the flow rate in mL/minute and drops per minute if 1 mL = 25 drops.

The answer is required in minutes, so it is necessary to convert the flow rate of milligrams per hour to milligrams per minute.
    Let the number of millilitres per minute be y. Setting up proportional sets:

mass of drug (mg)	2	y
time (minutes)	60	1

We can spot that 60 is divided by 30 to give 2, so 1 is divided by 30 to give y, therefore:

$y = 0.033$

The flow rate is 0.033 mg per minute.
    Now we need to find the volume of solution that contains 0.033 mg. We know that the solution contains 0.05 mg/mL.
    Let the volume of solution that contains 0.033 mg be x. Setting up proportional sets:

volume of solution (mL)	1	x
mass of drug (mg)	0.05	0.033

We can spot that 0.05 is divided by 0.05 to give 1, so 0.033 is divided by 0.05 to give x, therefore:

$x = 0.66$

0.66 mL of solution contains 0.033 mg of drug. Since the drug has to be given at the rate of 0.033 mg per minute, the correct flow rate for the drug solution is 0.66 mL per minute.

Given that 1 mL is equivalent to 25 drops, it is possible to convert 0.66 mL to drops.

Let the number of drops in 0.66 mL be z. Setting up proportional sets:

number of drops	25	z
volume (mL)	1	0.66

We can spot that 1 is multiplied by 25 to give 25, so 0.66 is multiplied by 25 to give z, therefore:

$z = 16.5$

The administration set should be adjusted to give 16.5 drops per minute.

Some solutions of drugs are required to be delivered continuously. In such a situation a syringe driver is used. The syringe driver is calibrated as the distance the driver moves per unit of time. It is therefore necessary to calculate the rate of delivery in order to give a known amount of drug.

EXAMPLE 9.7

Apomorphine injection may be given via a syringe driver with a rate setting in mm/hour. Apomorphine injection contains 10 mg apomorphine per millilitre. It is usual to dilute the injection with an equal volume of sodium chloride 0.9% before adding it to the 10 mL syringe. The 10 mL syringe has a length of 60 mm. If the patient requires 7.5 mg of apomorphine per hour, at what rate setting should the syringe driver be fixed?

First it is necessary to calculate the amount of drug contained in the

10 mL syringe. The apomorphine solution is prepared by mixing 5 mL of apomorphine injection with 5 mL of sodium chloride solution. 5 mL of apomorphine injection (10 mg/mL) contains 50 mg of apomorphine, and so there must be 50 mg of apomorphine in the 10 mL of solution. The patient requires 7.5 mg of apomorphine per hour and we know that 50 mg is contained in 10 mL. We also know that the 10 mL is contained in a syringe that is 60 mm in length. We therefore need to calculate the number of millimetres that will contain 7.5 mg.

Let the number of millimetres containing 7.5 mg be x. Setting up proportional sets:

length (mm)	60	x
mass of apomorphine (mg)	50	7.5

$$\frac{x}{7.5} = \frac{60}{50}$$

$$x = 60 \times \frac{7.5}{50}$$

$$x = 9$$

9 mm of the syringe contains 7.5 mg of apomorphine. If the patient is to receive 7.5 mg per hour, the syringe driver should be set at 9 mm per hour.

Isotonicity

Solutions of drugs that are placed in contact with mucous membranes may cause stinging, irritation and cell destruction. These effects can be minimised by making the solution isotonic with the mucous membrane.

Osmotic pressure is a property of ions or molecules dissolved in water. Freezing point depression is related to the ions or molecules dissolved in water. It is the relationship between freezing point depression and osmotic pressure that is used in the formulation of isotonic and iso-osmotic solutions.

A 0.9% w/v solution of sodium chloride in water is iso-osmotic and isotonic with blood, serum and other body fluids such as tears. In other words, it has the same osmotic pressure. 0.9% w/v sodium chloride solution freezes at −0.52°C and so do blood, serum and other body fluids. Other solutions that freeze at −0.52°C will therefore be isotonic with blood, serum, etc. A 0.9% w/v solution of sodium chloride is known as 'normal saline solution'.

A solution of a small amount of a drug in water will probably have an osmotic pressure less than that of body fluids. In order to make the solution isotonic, it is necessary to add another substance. The usual adjusting substance is sodium chloride, since it is found in body fluids and is non-toxic. A table of iso-osmotic concentrations and freezing point depressions for many drugs can be found in *The Pharmaceutical Codex*.

The proportional sets approach can be used to calculate the amount of adjusting substance required to be added to a solution in order to make it isotonic. However, the relationship between freezing point depression and concentration of the ion or molecule is not linear, although all methods of calculation assume a linear relationship over a small temperature range. In practice all solutions should be tested for isotonicity to ensure that the theoretical calculations (whatever method is used) are valid.

EXAMPLE 9.8

Calculate the amount of sodium chloride that should be added to the following formulation of nasal drops in order to make the final solution isotonic:

ephedrine hydrochloride	*0.5 g*
water to	*100 mL*

Note: A 1% w/v solution of ephedrine hydrochloride depresses the freezing point by 0.169°C and a 1% w/v solution of sodium chloride depresses the freezing point by 0.576°C. Remember that an isotonic solution freezes at –0.52°C.

It is necessary to calculate the freezing point depression attributable to the ephedrine hydrochloride (0.5 g in 100 mL = 0.5% w/v).

Let the freezing point depression caused by the ephedrine hydrochloride be x. Setting up proportional sets:

ephedrine hydrochloride (% w/v)	1	0.5
freezing point depression (°C)	0.169	x

$$\frac{x}{0.5} = \frac{0.169}{1}$$

$$x = 0.0845$$

The ephedrine hydrochloride depresses the freezing point to 0.0845° below 0°C, that is to −0.0845°C.

The added sodium chloride will be required to depress the freezing point of the ephedrine solution by a further 0.4355°C so that it reaches the isotonic solution freezing point of −0.52°C. The amount of sodium chloride required to be added to the ephedrine hydrochloride solution has to be calculated. Let the % w/v sodium chloride required to depress the freezing point by 0.4355°C be z.

Setting up proportional sets:

sodium chloride (% w/v)	1	z
freezing point depression (°C)	0.576	0.4355

$$\frac{z}{0.4355} = \frac{1}{0.576}$$

$$z = \frac{0.4355}{0.576}$$

$$z = 0.756$$

0.756% w/v of sodium chloride should be added to the formula to ensure the final solution is isotonic.

....

Practice calculations

Answers are given at the end of the chapter.

Q1   1 L of glucose 5% solution is to be given to a patient over a 5-hour period. Calculate the rate of delivery in mL/minute.

Q2   500 mL of normal saline solution is to be given to a patient over a 6-hour period. If 20 drops = 1 mL, calculate how many drops per minute should be administered to the patient.

Q3   An intravenous solution is to be administered at a rate of

2 mL/minute. What volume will be required if the infusion is to be maintained for 3 hours?

Q4   A 10 mL vial of multivitamin injection is to be added to 500 mL of glucose 5% solution. The resultant solution is to be administered to a patient over 3 hours. The administration set is calibrated at 20 drops/mL. Calculate the number of drops per minute to be given if the patient is to receive all the solution in the specified time.

Q5   Nizatidine injection (25 mg/mL) is supplied in 4 mL vials. The BNF states that for continuous infusion 'dilute 300 mg in 150 mL and give at a rate of 10 mg/hour'. If this procedure is adopted, calculate:

(a) how many vials of nizatidine injection will be required
(b) the flow rate (in mL/hour)
(c) the length of time the infusion will take.

Q6   A pharmacist prepares a solution of vancomycin containing 1 g in 200 mL. The rate of infusion should not exceed 10 mg/minute.

(a) Calculate the maximum flow rate in mL/minute.
(b) If the decision is to give the infusion over 2 hours, calculate the flow rate in mL/minute.

Q7   A baby weighing 3.4 kg requires treatment with phenytoin at a dose of 20 mg/kg. A 5 mL vial of phenytoin injection containing 50 mg/mL is available for dilution prior to infusion. A suitable volume of phenytoin injection is diluted up to 50 mL with sodium chloride 0.9%.

(a) Calculate the volume of phenytoin injection that must be used in the preparation of the infusion.
(b) The infusion rate must not exceed 3 mg/kg/minute. Calculate the maximum flow rate in mL/minute if these conditions are applied to the administration.
(c) The infusion must be completed in 1 hour. Calculate the minimum flow rate (in mL/minute) if the infusion is completed in 1 hour.

Q8   The recommended dose of drug X is 75 mg by slow infusion at a rate not exceeding 0.3 g/hour. Drug X is available as an injection containing 15 mg of drug X in 1 mL. Calculate the volume of drug X injection required and the infusion rate in mL/minute.

Q9 A drug is provided as an infusion solution at a concentration of 2 micrograms per millilitre. The prescribed flow rate is 0.05 mg per hour. Calculate the flow rate in mL/minute and drops per minute if 1 mL = 25 drops.

Q10 A syringe driver is designed to contain 5 mL of injection and has a length of 60 mm. Injection Y contains 4 mg/mL. If a patient requires 2.5 mg of drug Y per hour, at what rate setting in mm/hour should the syringe driver be fixed?

Q11 A syringe driver is set at 5 mm/hour. The length of the syringe driver is 80 mm and it holds 10 mL of injection solution. An injection solution contains 5 micrograms of drug X in 1 mL. What dose of drug X will the syringe driver deliver in 3 hours?

Q12 An intravenous solution of sodium chloride 0.2% requires to be made isotonic by the addition of anhydrous glucose. What weight of anhydrous glucose is required in the preparation of 1 L of the intravenous solution?
(A 1% solution of sodium chloride depresses the freezing point of water by 0.576°C. A 1% solution of anhydrous glucose depresses the freezing point of water by 0.1037°C.)

Q13 Zinc sulphate 0.25% eye drops are required to be made isotonic with sodium chloride. What weight of sodium chloride is required in the preparation of 100 mL of eye-drop solution?
(A 0.25% solution of zinc sulphate depresses the freezing point of water by 0.022°C.)

Q14 How much sodium chloride should be added in the preparation of 25 mL of pilocarpine hydrochloride 2% eye drops to render them isotonic?
(A 2% solution of pilocarpine hydrochloride depresses the freezing point of water by 0.262°C.)

Q15 Using the information in question 14, explain why it may not be possible or necessary to make pilocarpine hydrochloride 4% eye drops isotonic.

Q16 How much sodium chloride is required in the preparation of 50 mL of isotonic amethocaine hydrochloride 0.5% solution? Assume the sodium chloride is used for isotonicity adjustment only.
(A 0.5% solution of amethocaine hydrochloride depresses the freezing point of water by 0.062°C.)

Answers

A1 3.33 mL/minute

A2 28 drops per minute

A3 360 mL

A4 56.6 drops per minute

A5 (a) 3 vials
(b) 5 mL/hour
(c) 30 hours

A6 (a) 2 mL/minute
(b) 1.66 mL/minute

A7 (a) 1.36 mL
(b) 7.5 mL/minute
(c) 0.833 mL/minute

A8 5 mL
0.33 mL/minute

A9 0.417 mL/minute
10.4 drops per minute

A10 7.5 mm/hour

A11 9.357 micrograms

A12   39.03 g

A13   0.864 g

A14   0.112 g

A15   The depression due to 4% pilocarpine hydrochloride is 0.524°C, which is about the same as that of an isotonic solution.

A16   0.398 g

Bibliography

British National Formulary, current edition. London: British Medical Association and Royal Pharmaceutical Society of Great Britain (published biannually in March and September).

British Pharmacopeia, current edition. London: HMSO (updated annually).

Martindale: The complete drug reference, 32nd edn (Parfitt K, ed.). London: Pharmaceutical Press, 1999.

Medicines, Ethics and Practice. London: Pharmaceutical Press (published biannually in January and July).

The Pharmaceutical Codex: Principles and practice of pharmaceutics, 12th edn (Lund W, ed.). London: Pharmaceutical Press, 1994.

Appendix: Atomic weights of the elements ($^{12}C = 12$)

Atomic number	Name	Symbol	Atomic weight
89	Actinium	Ac	*
13	Aluminium	Al	26.981 538
95	Americium	Am	*
51	Antimony	Sb	121.760
18	Argon	Ar	39.948
33	Arsenic	As	74.92 160
85	Astatine	At	*
56	Barium	Ba	137.327
97	Berkelium	Bk	*
4	Beryllium	Be	9.012 182
83	Bismuth	Bi	208.98 038
107	Bohrium	Bh	*
5	Boron	B	10.811
35	Bromine	Br	79.904
48	Cadmium	Cd	112.411
55	Caesium	Cs	132.90 545
20	Calcium	Ca	40.078
98	Californium	Cf	*
6	Carbon	C	12.0107
58	Cerium	Ce	140.116
17	Chlorine	Cl	35.4527
24	Chromium	Cr	51.9961
27	Cobalt	Co	58.933 200
29	Copper	Cu	63.546
96	Curium	Cm	*
105	Dubnium	Db	*
66	Dysprosium	Dy	162.50
99	Einsteinium	Es	*
68	Erbium	Er	167.26
63	Europium	Eu	151.964
100	Fermium	Fm	*
9	Fluorine	F	18.9 984 032
87	Francium	Fr	*
64	Gadolinium	Gd	157.25

Atomic number	Name	Symbol	Atomic weight
31	Gallium	Ga	69.723
32	Germanium	Ge	72.61
79	Gold	Au	196.96 655
72	Hafnium	Hf	178.49
108	Hassium	Hs	*
2	Helium	He	4.002 602
67	Holmium	Ho	164.93 032
1	Hydrogen	H	1.00 794
49	Indium	In	114.818
53	Iodine	I	126.90 447
77	Iridium	Ir	192.217
26	Iron	Fe	55.845
36	Krypton	Kr	83.80
57	Lanthanum	La	138.9 055
103	Lawrencium	Lr	*
82	Lead	Pb	207.2
3	‡Lithium	Li	6.941
71	Lutetium	Lu	174.967
12	Magnesium	Mg	24.3050
25	Manganese	Mn	54.938 049
109	Meitnerium	Mt	*
101	Mendelevium	Md	*
80	Mercury	Hg	200.59
42	Molybdenum	Mo	95.94
60	Neodymium	Nd	144.24
10	Neon	Ne	20.1797
93	Neptunium	Np	*
28	Nickel	Ni	58.6934
41	Niobium	Nb	92.90 638
7	Nitrogen	N	14.00 674
102	Nobelium	No	*
76	Osmium	Os	190.23
8	Oxygen	O	15.9994
46	Palladium	Pd	106.42
15	Phosphorus	P	30.973 761
78	Platinum	Pt	195.078
94	Plutonium	Pu	*
84	Polonium	Po	*
19	Potassium	K	39.0983
59	Praseodymium	Pr	140.90 765
61	Promethium	Pm	*
91	†Protactinium	Pa	231.03 588
88	Radium	Ra	*
86	Radon	Rn	*
75	Rhenium	Re	186.207

Atomic number	Name	Symbol	Atomic weight
45	Rhodium	Rh	102.90 550
37	Rubidium	Rb	85.4678
44	Ruthenium	Ru	101.07
104	Rutherfordium	Rf	*
62	Samarium	Sm	150.36
21	Scandium	Sc	44.955 910
106	Seaborgium	Sg	*
34	Selenium	Se	78.96
14	Silicon	Si	28.0855
47	Silver	Ag	107.8682
11	Sodium	Na	22.989 770
38	Strontium	Sr	87.62
16	Sulphur	S	32.066
73	Tantalum	Ta	180.9479
43	Technetium	Tc	*
52	Tellurium	Te	127.60
65	Terbium	Tb	158.92 534
81	Thallium	Tl	204.3833
90	†Thorium	Th	232.0381
69	Thulium	Tm	168.93 421
50	Tin	Sn	118.710
22	Titanium	Ti	47.867
74	Tungsten	W	183.84
110	Ununnilium	Uun	*
111	Unununium	Uuu	*
92	†Uranium	U	238.0289
23	Vanadium	V	50.9415
54	Xenon	Xe	131.29
70	Ytterbium	Yb	173.04
39	Yttrium	Y	88.90 585
30	Zinc	Zn	65.39
40	Zirconium	Zr	91.224

Elements marked * have no stable nuclides and IUPAC states 'there is no general agreement on which of the isotopes of the radioactive elements is, or is likely to be judged "important" and various criteria such as "longest half-life", "production in quantity", "used commercially", etc., have been applied in the Commission's choice.' However, atomic weights are given for radioactive elements marked † as they do have a characteristic terrestrial isotopic composition. Commercially available lithium (‡) materials have atomic weights ranging from 6.94 to 6.99; if a more accurate value is required, it must be determined for the specific material.

Index

Tables are indicated in *italic* type

accuracy
  in arithmetic calculations   12
  measurement   9
age, for dosage calculation   *114, 119, 121*
alcohol, example of mixing different strengths   85
amount strength
  units   44
  examples   *44–45*
anhydrates of drugs   158–160
aromatic waters *see* concentrated waters
atomic weight   151, 197–199

body surface area, for dosage calculation   *119*
body weight, for dosage calculation   *114*
bulk density   136

centigrade *see* Celsius; temperature, Celsius
children's doses *see* dose
chloroform water
  concentrate   67–68
  see also concentrated waters
concentrated waters
  chloroform water   66
  peppermint water   66
  rose water   66
concentration
  amount strengths   44
  calculating amounts for known percentage solution   54
  calculating for ratio strength solution   55
  converting expressions   49–54
  mixing two known concentrations   81–87
  parts per million   47–48

percentage concentration   49
ratio strengths   45–46
conversions
  Celsius to Fahrenheit and vice versa   37–39
  decimals
    to fractions   7
    to percentages   8
  expressions of concentration   49–54
  fractions to percentages   8
  volume to weight   143
  weight to volume   144

decimals   6
  conversion
    to fractions   7
    to percentage   8
  correction
    to decimal places   11
    to significant figures   11
  place values   6
degree of accuracy   9
degrees, Celsius *see* temperature
degrees, Fahrenheit *see* temperature
denominator *see* fractions
density   143–145
dilutions   61–86
  mixing two known concentrations   81–87
  serial   63–66
  simple   61–63
displacement values   136–143
displacement volumes   131–135
  for powder injections   *133*
dosage regimen   105
dose
  body surface area and   118
  body weight and   113
  daily   105
  daily divided   105

liquid formulations and   108, 111
  as a percentage of adult dose   120
  single   105
  solid formulations and   106, 110
  total   105
  units and   121
  units of formulation and   106
  weekly   105
  weight of drug and   110
drops, delivery from parenteral
          solutions *see* parenteral solutions

empirical formula   152
errors, build-up in arithmetic
          calculations   12

Fahrenheit *see* temperature
flow rate *see* rate of flow
formulations
  increasing the formula   93–94
  involving parts   94–97
  involving percentages   97–99
  reducing the formula   91–93
fractions
  conversion
      to decimals   7
      to percentage   8
  denominator   3–4
  expressed in their lowest form   5
  multiplied by whole number   6
  numerator   3–4
freezing point
  calculation of isotonic solutions
          189–190
  blood, serum etc.   188
freezing point depression   189–190

gram   33
gram equivalent   173–174
glyco gelatin suppository base   140–142

height, for dosage calculation   114
hydrates of drugs   159–160

injections   113, 131–134, 157
integer   6
intravenous solutions *see* parenteral
          solutions
iso-osmotic solutions   188
isotonic solutions *see* isotonicity
isotonicity   188–190

kilo *see* metric units
kilogram   33

legal classification of drugs   162–165
  based on
      maximum dose (calculated as
          base)   162
      maximum strength of base   163
      maximum strength and maximum
          dose   164
litre   33

mass   33
  see also weight
mega *see* metric units
method
  A *see* proportional sets
  B *see* proportional sets
  C *see* proportional sets
metric units   33
  conversion
      one metric unit to another   34–35
      metric to non-metric units and vice
          versa   36–37
  kilo   34
  micro   34
  milli   34
  mega   34
micro *see* metric units
micromole   166
milli *see* metric units
milliequivalents   173–175
millimoles   165–169
molar solutions   169–173
molecular weight   151–175
  see also legal classification
moles   165–169

nanomoles   166
natural number *see* number
newtons   33
number
  natural   3
  rational   3
  treatment days   107
numerator *see* fractions

ointments   96–99, 144–146
oral syringe   109
osmotic pressure   188
  adjustment with sodium chloride   189

paediatric doses *see* dose
parenteral solutions   179–188
  see also rate of flow
parts *see* formulations

parts per million
  definition   47
  examples   47–48
peppermint water *see* concentrated
    waters
percentage
  concentration
    definition   49
    examples   49
  definition   8
  conversion
    decimal to percentage   8
    fraction to percentage   8
pessary
  calculations   136
  calibration of mould   137
  glyco gelatin base   141
picomole   166
pints   36
place values *see* decimals
pounds   36
powder calculations   70–75
ppm *see* parts per million
proportional   1
proportional sets
  determination
    method A   15
    method B   16
    method C   17
  finding a missing value from   14
  of numbers   1–3
  setting up   21–24
  spot or spotting   16–17
  trivial   25

rate of flow
  amount of drug delivered over
      specified time period   183–188
  volume delivered over specific time
      period   179–183
ratio strengths
  definition   45
  examples   45–47
  units   43
rational number *see* numbers
ratios   3
rose water *see* concentrated waters

salts of drugs   154–161
  calculating weight
    if drug expressed as base   156–158

equivalent to known weight of
    base   158–159
serial dilution *see* dilutions
SI *see* Système International
significant figures   10
  correction
    to specific number of decimal
        places   11–12
    to fewer significant figures   11
spotting *see* proportional sets
stock solutions   63
simple dilutions *see* dilutions
stones   36
structural formula   152
suppositories
  calculations   136
  glyco gelatin base   140
  nominal sizes   137
  waxy/oily bases   137
suppository moulds, calibration   137
syringe driver   187–188
Système International   33

temperature
  Celsius   37–39
  conversions between Celsius and
      Fahrenheit   37–39
  Fahrenheit   37–39
  see also freezing point; freezing point
      depression
theobroma oil suppository base
    137–140
triturations   68–70
  powders   71–75

v/v *see* volume in volume
v/w *see* volume in weight
valency   174
volume in volume   43
volume in weight   43

w/v *see* weight in volume
w/w *see* weight in weight
water of crystallisation   168
  see also hydrates of drugs
waxy/oily suppository base   137–140
weight   33
  see also mass
weight in volume   33, 43
  see also density
weight in weight   33, 43